7722   616·0472 H6A   10093
$\times$ £25·00

|

)

OXFORD MEDICAL PUBLICATIONS

PATIENT-CONTROLLED ANALGESIA

PATIENT-CONTROLLED ANALGESIA

Confidence in Postoperative Pain Control

MARGARET L. HEATH

*Consultant Anaesthetist, Lewisham
Hospital; Recognized Teacher
UMDS (Guy's Campus) University
of London*

VERONICA J. THOMAS

*Lecturer in Health Psychology
and Nursing Studies, Department of
Nursing Studies, Kings College, University of London*

Oxford   New York   Tokyo
OXFORD UNIVERSITY PRESS
1993

Oxford University Press, Walton Street, Oxford OX2 6DP

Oxford New York Toronto
Delhi Bombay Calcutta Madras Karachi
Kuala Lumpur Singapore Hong Kong Tokyo
Nairobi Dar es Salaam Cape Town
Melbourne Auckland Madrid
and associated companies in
Berlin Ibadan

Oxford is a trade mark of Oxford University Press

Published in the United States
by Oxford University Press Inc., New York

A catalogue record for this book is available from the British Library

Library of Congress Cataloging in Publication Data
Heath, Margaret L. (Margaret Longden)
Patient controlled analgesia: confidence in postoperative pain
control/Margaret L. Heath, Veronica J. Thomas.
Includes bibliographical references.
1. Patient-contolled analgesia. 2. Postoperative pain-
Chemotherapy. I. Thomas, Veronica J. II. Title.
{DNLM: 1. Analgesia, Patient-Controlled. 2. Pain, Postoperative-
drug therapy. WO 184 H438p 1993}
RD98.4.H43 1993 616'.0472–dc20 93–1605
ISBN 0–19–262165–3

Typeset by The Electronic Book Factory Ltd, Fife. Scotland.
Printed in Great Britain by
Bookcraft (Bath) Ltd

Preface

Patient-controlled analgesia has been possible for over twenty years. Despite its enthusiastic acceptance by those patients and staff with experience, it has yet to become widely available as a routine method of postoperative pain control. Recent changes make it seem possible that this can now happen: acceptable technology is available, and improvement in postoperative pain relief has been called for publicly by surgeons and anaesthetists; in addition, the patient's voice may become more audible as the NHS evolves.

This book is designed to help all those concerned with enabling patients to benefit from PCA—anaesthetists, recovery staff, ward nurses, surgical residents, and pharmacists, whether or not they are members of dedicated Acute Pain Teams. Understanding pain is as important as understanding the drugs and equipment, and we hope the book will also be of value to senior students of medicine and nursing.

London   M.L.H.
May 1993   V.J.T.

Contents

1 Introduction

Surgical operations are almost inevitably followed by pain which assaults the patient as the anaesthetic wears off. Whilst it must be acknowledged that some of the problems of postoperative pain are insoluble for basic physiological reasons, the degree of pain and suffering is frequently disproportionate to the trauma. Many researchers, doctors, and patients have drawn attention to the unsatisfactory nature of this situation, which was well summarized by a joint working party of the Royal College of Surgeons and the College of Anaesthetists in their 1990 report *Pain after surgery*.

As there is already a wide range of potent, effective narcotic agents, the focus of attention in addressing this problem has been turned away from the search for the perfect drug and has concentrated on the need to provide optimal methods of analgesic administration. To this end, researchers have concentrated on a need to integrate drug-based knowledge with the response of the individual patient to the drugs. Whilst these are important elements of any pain-relief system one further factor must be added: the personal experience of the patient. We have chosen in this book to focus on Patient-Controlled Analgesia (PCA), a method which depends on all three elements. It combines effectiveness with patient safety and adds little to the complexity of care, requiring no changes in the normal progression of the patient through the recovery area and back to the ward. PCA's promotion of recovery can in part be attributed to physiological factors: the ability to maintain optimum plasma concentrations with the minimum of drug. In addition, the speed of onset reduces the overall period of distress, and thus may relieve anxiety. Its most important feature, however, and that which sets it apart from other methods, is its requirement for active participation by the patient. Therefore the importance of the patient's psychology in contributing to its usefulness is given full significance, as is recommended in the report alluded to above.

Traditional regimes have greatly underestimated this facet, despite the wealth of research demonstrating that emotional and personality factors influence the experience of postoperative pain. These sources have reinforced our own research and experience, and have led us to emphasize in this book the importance of psychological factors in postoperative pain-experience, and to highlight their relevance to PCA.

We have sought to provide a thorough grounding in the practical aspects as well as the psychology and pharmacology, and to support our views wherever possible with relevant research findings. Although PCA will normally be set up by the anaesthetist, the understanding and involvement of recovery and ward nurses and surgical house officers is vital if the patient is to reap the maximum possible benefits (both physical and psychological) that contribute so much to postoperative recovery. Pharmacists can also play a substantial role in both the technical and clinical aspects. All staff, in their turn, will gain increased satisfaction from contributing to improved care.

We have restricted ourselves to the intravenous (IV) route, although the principle of patient control can be extended to other delivery routes, notably the epidural. The benefits and dangers of these other regimes require further evaluation.

In the 1970s labour wards in the UK underwent a transformation in atmosphere and in attitudes to pain when epidural analgesia found its place as a safe and effective technique. We believe that patient-controlled analgesia can bring about a similar transformation in postoperative care in our hospitals during the 1990s. Although many aspects require further research, sufficient investigation and development of the technique has been undertaken to convince us that there should be no further delay in its widespread adoption. The effectiveness of research findings in changing everyday practice is notorious for its variability; this book is intended to support surgical care teams in the practical and philosophical transition from regimes that are unsatisfactory for both patients and themselves to a patient-centred approach that can transform the postoperative period.

We cannot ignore the immense changes that have taken place within the UK National Health Service as a result of economic pressures. Patterns of care have changed: in particular there has been a remarkable reduction in the length of in-patient stay for the majority of conditions. The reduction in length of postoperative stay is almost entirely beneficial to patients, although the overall intensity of in-patient care has thereby increased, with consequent heavy pressure on all staff. We have tried to take account of these realities, and are thankful that the regimes that we advocate can contribute effectively to the quality of patient care without adding to the net burden on staff or resources.

We admit freely that PCA was introduced somewhat haphazardly into Lewisham Hospital, with each anaesthetist taking individual responsibility. Despite many determined efforts and the expenditure of a great deal of time and energy we have yet to achieve our aim of having all medical and nursing staff understanding the underlying basis, nor have sufficient staff been trained in caring for patients on PCA to form a self-perpetuating core of experienced people. We confess to this to encourage others who may similarly have insufficient resources to set up a full Acute Pain Team, or who may encounter other difficulties along the way. Other hospitals have done much better, and we refer to their reports throughout this book. However, despite our inadequacies, PCA has been both safe and successful, and we now have adequate protocols and policies. We have little doubt that more patients could and will benefit, although many who have received PCA could have had even better pain relief with fewer side-effects if we had managed better training, supervision, and support.

2 Aims of perioperative care

All members of the team caring for patients requiring surgery need, occasionally, to spend a few moments reminding themselves of the basic objectives of their work. It is not the normal province of anyone except the surgeon to decide on the appropriate intervention; but every member of the team has a duty to consider whether further discussion and consultation might improve the quality of management, often from the point of view of timing, of preoperative preparation, or even of the extent of surgery. The contribution of the General Practitioner is clearly crucial in the early phase; but all members of the team can contribute.

Patients seek help primarily because they have identified some abnormality, and good care is directed towards:

- ensuring that the patient is optimally prepared physically and emotionally, given the time available;
- providing safe, efficient care during anaesthesia and surgery;
- minimizing the effects of physical and emotional trauma; and
- returning the patient as rapidly and as far as possible to independent, full function.

Box 1. Aims of perioperative care

1. Optimal preparation
2. Safe anaesthesia and surgery
3. Minimal adverse effects
4. Rapid, maximal return to normality

It must be recognized that fulfilling the latter two requirements will be greatly eased by effective application of the first two; indeed, to some extent, the overlap and interaction amongst all the factors become more obvious when it is realized that few patients are lucky enough to get away with only one operation in their lives: their first experience can have an immense effect on subsequent ones.

Equally, the natural optimism of people working in acute hospitals tends to make them treat everyone as if complete and perfect cure is the natural outcome of every episode. Patients are often much more realistic: many of them have more experience of disease—particularly their own—than the young staff with whom they are in most immediate contact. The professionals have the immense advantage of a wide, systematic knowledge of basic physiology and the common patterns of illness. This acts as a frame of reference and aids some sort of logical interpretation of events. Their judgement and skills will mature more quickly if they recognize and value the individual personal experience of each patient. A person can be thought of as a unique blend of physical and psychological factors interacting with the social environment. Even the most commonplace illness will be modified by these special characteristics of the individual.

It is a paradox that this approach is increasingly recognized as valuable at a time when great effort is being directed at minimizing in-patient care. It is the attitude that matters; large amounts of time are not necessary: good use of contact time is.

GENERAL FEATURES OF IMMEDIATE PREOPERATIVE CARE

The patient's needs

Mentally, patients need to know what to expect and to feel confident that those looking after them understand their present condition and any other medical and social facts that are relevant. Physically, the discomforts of preoperative investigation, restriction of oral intake, and simply having to wait around should be reduced in real terms as far as possible; their impact can also be appreciably diminished by helping patients to understand why there is a need for them.

The surgeon's needs

The surgeon's requirements are to a large extent organizational: a patient anaesthetized ready for operation at the planned time, whose preoperative workup has ensured as far as possible that the planned operation is the correct one.

The anaesthetist's needs

Briefly, the anaesthetist hopes for a patient in the best mental and physical state possible in the time available. There is an inevitable tension between exhaustive investigation and treatment of abnormalities that may prejudice safety and the relative urgency of the operation.

Each aspect of immediate preoperative care points up the need for the earlier, pre-hospital, phase. Screening of patients for incidental conditions which may be asymptomatic (for example diabetes and hypertension), for controllable risk factors such as obesity and smoking, and for recollection of adverse reactions to anaesthetics or other drugs can eliminate the disaster of last-minute cancellation. Cancellation is a disaster for the patient (time off work, someone to look after the children), the hospital (expensive theatre time wasted), and for all staff involved, who suffer a wide range of stress.

Each care team has to make its own decisions about routines and protocols. This should be a conscious process of consensus decision-making. To a certain extent, routines can free the mind from a weight of fairly petty decisions: every adult patient will have a bath and come to theatre wearing an operating gown and lying on a trolley, etc.; every patient over a certain age will have a preoperative ECG. However, insistence on over-complex routines can become depersonalizing to the point of barbarity—all in the name of safety: for instance, deaf patients should not be deprived of their hearing-aids until the last possible moment. Good information systems to ensure that the relevant staff know that the patient has an aid and that it does not get lost are what is needed. The Appendix to this chapter shows one approach to integrating preoperative preparation. The link between such matters and postoperative pain relief may seem somewhat tenuous: we think otherwise. Patient autonomy is vital to reduction in anxiety. As we stress repeatedly elsewhere in this book, successful management of pain depends on much more than giving drugs—even in the best available way. At a purely practical level, the example chosen above can make all the difference to successful communication with the patient in the recovery room. Even within teams that lay emphasis on providing good information for patients, too little attention is often given to following up with 'hard copy'. Written information with admirable content may indeed be available, but its style and presentation make it hard work even for the literate. Our children's wards have given an excellent lead with bright, boldly illustrated folders covering most common conditions. Words are few, simple, and large—ostensibly for the children; but covert observation has shown that parents also appreciate the style (Fig. 2.1.a). The advertising industry does not try to communicate with the public by issuing what look like extracts from textbooks (Fig. 2.1.b.).

Although information packs are primarily designed with patients for elective/scheduled surgery in mind, every attempt should be made to offer appropriate information to patients admitted unexpectedly (urgent or emergency cases). It is particularly important that care is taken postoperatively to make up for any deficiencies.

Box 2. Preoperative care for elective/scheduled surgery

Pre-admission: Information, decision-making

Investigation: ● specific to surgical procedure

● specific to age, previous history, medication

Immediately before operation: evaluation ● surgical

● anaesthetic

● nursing

information tailored to individual

Information related specifically to patient-controlled analgesia is considered in Chapter 5.

CARE DURING THE OPERATIVE PROCEDURE

Safe and efficient care during the operative procedure depend on both the surgical and the anaesthetic teams, whose skills are often taken for granted. The education and training of each member (medical and non-medical) of these teams require constant attention, and must be seen as dynamic processes, evolving as a result of experience and, most importantly, of the findings of well-founded research at all levels. The current obsession with efficiency must not be allowed to obscure this wider picture. Reduction in the underpinning of research and education is a form of asset-stripping that can make

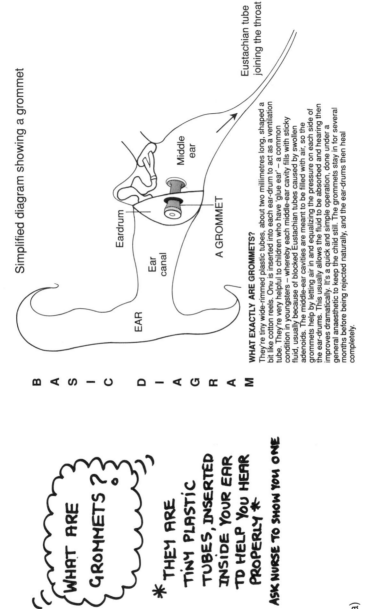

Simplified diagram showing a grommet

EAR

Ear
canal

Eardrum

Middle
ear

Eustachian tube
joining the throat

A GROMMET

WHAT EXACTLY ARE GROMMETS?
They're tiny wide-rimmed plastic tubes, about two millimetres long, shaped a
bit like cotton reels. One is inserted into each ear-drum to act as a ventilation
tube. They're very helpful to children who have 'glue ear' – a common
condition in youngsters – whereby each middle-ear cavity fills with sticky
fluid, usually because of blocked Eustachian tubes caused by swollen
adenoids. The middle-ear cavities are meant to be filled with air, so the
grommets help by letting air in and equalizing the pressure on each side of
the ear-drums. This usually allows the fluid to be absorbed and hearing then
improves dramatically. It's a quick and simple operation, done under a
general anaesthetic to keep the child still. The grommets stay in for several
months before being rejected naturally, and the ear-drums then heal
completely.

WHAT ARE
GROMMETS?

* THEY ARE
TINY PLASTIC
TUBES, INSERTED
INSIDE YOUR EAR
TO HELP YOU HEAR
PROPERLY *

ASK NURSE TO SHOW YOU ONE

(a)

Fig. 2.1. Two contrasting ways of presenting information to patients: (a) sheet from a children's information folder, Lewisham Hospital; (b) information handout sheet on postoperative care from the Day Surgical Unit, Lewisham Hospital.

CARE FOLLOWING A HERNIA OPERATION

It is important that you read and follow these instructions carefully to prevent any complications after your operation. If you have any questions, do not hesitate to ask a nurse or doctor.

CARE OF THE WOUND

The wound should be kept as dry as possible until initial healing has taken place and the wound has been inspected by a nurse or doctor (sometimes there is slight oozing from the wound and a dry pad is placed over the wound). The area around the wound may itch and you may also experience a numb patch around the wound. The scar may be red and prominent after the stitches have been removed—this will fade gradually. The scar may be softened by gently rubbing in a lanolin cream or 'Nivea'. If you are worried about the condition of your wound, do not hesitate to contact your doctor.

YOUR RECOVERY AND DISCHARGE HOME

You must appreciate that even though your hernia has been repaired it will still be months before it is safe to carry out most normal 'straining' activities you were doing before. Even though your wound looks healed on the surface, deep inside there will be a weakness for a while. It is important therefore not to **STRAIN** the wound.

1. PAIN

   Our object is to prevent or minimize pain by offering you regular painkillers in the form of an injection initially or tablets, e.g. Paracetamol. These will help take away the 'soreness' from the 'cut' and any general throbbing-type pain, enabling you to move and cough more easily.

2. COUGH

   We advise you to give up smoking prior to your operation and to inform your doctor if you have a chesty cough so that it can be relieved before the operation. When coughing immediately after the operation it is helpful if you support your wound by holding it with your hands, to ensure you cough up any sputum properly to avoid a chest infection. If you develop a cough take a mixture to soothe your throat and help you expectorate.

3. BOWELS

   Ensure that you do not get constipated, as this will strain your wound. You will probably not have your bowels open until at least 2 days after the operation. Take a high-fibre diet or a regular laxative if required.

4. GETTING AROUND

   You must walk around as naturally as possible after the operation. Once home you must take regular exercise by walking, but avoid running or strenuous exercise.

5. LIFTING

   Do not carry or lift heavy items for about 3 months—e.g. heavy suitcase, vacuum cleaner.

6. DISCHARGE

   You will be discharged home on the same day—the day of the operation. You should have someone to escort you home and look after you at home.

7. RETURNING TO WORK

   This does depend on what your job is. Please discuss this with your doctor. It is advisable to remain off work for at least 3 weeks if you have a sedentary job, e.g. office work, or for a longer period if you have a more strenuous labouring job.

8. DRIVING

   It is not advisable to drive for at least 3 weeks, and do not drive on long journeys for 3 months.

9. FOLLOW-UP

   An appointment will be required, and this will be made prior to your discharge; the length of time depends on your condition.

a very short-term saving at the expense of the destruction of the future of health care within the UK.

Appropriate equipment, both surgical and anaesthetic, has proved less of a problem to obtain than to manage; but standards of checking and maintenance have steadily improved, and few clinicians should now feel severely restricted in this area. The operative period is rightly regarded as so important that serious deficiencies are rare. Patients can be confident that procedures will be both safe and effective.

Box 3. Operative care

Resource	**Back-up**
Trained staff ● medical	Continuing education
● non-medical	and training
Equipment—	Maintenance and replacement
selected, commissioned	programme

THE IMMEDIATE RECOVERY PERIOD

Not very long ago, the immediate recovery period was longer and much less well supervised than is now the rule; it was commonplace for patients to be collected directly from the theatre by a ward nurse and to return to the ward before they had regained control of the airway. Accidents were frequent. Recent studies of perioperative mortality (Lunn and Mushin 1982; Buck *et al*. 1989) show that few patients die within this time now, but that there are difficulties in maintaining the same standard of care round the clock: many hospitals do not keep recovery areas staffed at nights or weekends (Dowie 1991). Restricting the number of sites offering continuous operating facilities may be better for patients than allowing substandard care in a large number of units.

Originally introduced to allow airway and respiratory supervision, the recovery room rapidly became the place where cardiovascular stability and fluid balance were checked. Soon, the idea of administering the first dose of opiate was seen to be attractive. However, the intramuscular route demanded a safety period to try to ensure that the full effects of the dose, mainly possible respiratory depression, would be seen before the journey back to the ward. Efficacy was rarely evaluated, and the common rule that patients had to remain for 30 minutes after an injection meant that a busy nurse would prefer to get the patient back to the ward without 'post-op'. Thus the golden opportunity to control pain before the patient experienced its full severity was frequently missed.

Anaesthetists involved in chronic pain therapy have long realized the importance of preventing patients being overwhelmed by pain. The same outlook has only just started to prevail in the treatment of acute pain. The crucial role of the recovery area in ensuring a smooth transition from anaesthesia to appropriate pain control must become more firmly established, and this will reinforce the need for fully staffed recovery facilities for every surgical patient.

Box 4. Functions of Recovery facilities

- Close monitoring
- Post-anaesthetic care: for example, airway
- Post-surgical care: for example, fluid therapy
- Pain assessment and control

THE FIRST FEW DAYS

The majority of operations interfere with full function, cause pain, and require healing processes in direct proportion to their magnitude and severity. The interaction of these features is often not fully appreciated. Pain can inhibit a wide variety of functions, and restriction of movement can be particularly harmful, because thromboses and chest infections are thereby encouraged. Many aspects of recovery, including nutrition, blood-flow, oxygenation of tissues, and mobilization leading to maintenance or restoration of muscle mass can be improved by good pain control.

However, at the other end of the scale, some minor operations can be disproportionately painful, and, although the pain may be very short-lived, much suffering can be alleviated by prompt treatment directed at the patient's experience rather than any preconceived idea about how much pain relief 'should' be required in any particular circumstance.

Effective, safe treatment of severe acute pain has, in the past, been regarded as an expensive optional extra, requiring extra staff and equipment and carrying inevitable penalties of sedation or respiratory depression. More recently, research and experience have come to replace that view with one that sees good pain control as a cost-effective strategy for improving postoperative recovery.

Box 5. Post-Recovery Room care

- Mobilization
- Restoration of function and independence
- Nutrition
- Assessment and control of pain

APPENDIX: PRE-ANAESTHETIC CARE AND PREPARATION

A policy statement for nursing and medical staff from:
The Anaesthetic Department of Lewisham Hospital

General philosophy

Every patient to be cared for by the anaesthetic department will be visited by an anaesthetist, who will normally be one of the team scheduled to provide care.

On admission

In the time before this visit much can be done that is helpful: the more a patient understands his/her condition, the less anxiety is generated, the less analgesia is needed postoperatively, and the quicker is recovery. Parents and other relatives should be involved in this process whenever appropriate. It is very important, however, that confusing statements are not made: unless you are sure of your information use general statements ('our anaesthetists use the methods best suited to each condition; modern drugs and equipment ensure that you are looked after in the best way / are made as pain-free as possible after operation; the anaesthetist will explain the details and will welcome your interest').

Please feel free to draw our attention to any aspect of the patient's personal, social, or medical details: nurses and housemen are in the best position to pick up hints about odd drug reactions in the past, vague (or specific) fears about anaesthetic mishaps, or worries about postoperative pain.

Postoperatively

We will try to visit everyone postop, but this is the aspect that gets squeezed out when we are too busy: **please help us by contacting the anaesthetic department if anything has happened that you or the patient feel should not have done.** It is very important that the patient is taken seriously however bizarre the complaint may seem.

Nursing preparation

Record weight and results of urine test.

Oral intake

Unless the patient's surgical condition dictates otherwise, fluids should be unrestricted up to 4 hours before premedication time (5 hours before scheduled list-start time if no premed time written). A light, fat-free meal may also be taken up to this time; but heavy, fatty food should not be taken within six hours of premedication.

If the anaesthetist wishes a particular patient to be allowed or encouraged to drink after this time, specific instructions will be written in consultation with nursing staff.

Drugs

All prescribed medicines should be given as charted. A reasonable amount of water (e.g. 60 ml) can be allowed for swallowing any tablets.

If the anaesthetists wish any drug to be omitted they will place a cross in the appropriate square on the prescription chart. 'NIL BY MOUTH' does not apply to medication.

Dental prostheses

Should be noted and removed at premedication time; specific instructions will be written if they are NOT to be removed. **Other prostheses and hearing aids** should be noted but NOT

REMOVED unless specific instructions are given. Any patients who are very dependent on their glasses should keep them on; if possible, a case for them should be brought to theatre.

Journey to theatre

Most patients are put on to a canvas for lifting purposes; please ensure that it is laid so that the top edge is level with the top of the mattress—this ensures that the head is safely supported if the patient is lifted whilst unconscious. Patients should have as many pillows as they need to be comfortable. Unpremedicated patients may walk to theatre if they prefer; children may be carried.

Medical preparation

The aim of pre-anaesthetic care by other medical staff should be to get the patient as fit as possible in the time available. The time available depends on the urgency of the operation: we will anaesthetize patients who are desperately sick if that is in their best interests, but we will be very fussy about patients having minor, non-essential operations—if anything goes wrong we have to feel able to face the patient, their relatives, our peers, and even the coroner.

We need the results of all investigations done prior to admission as well as those you order (checking the notes often reveals that sickle screen and blood group have been previously determined). In addition, please help us by:

1. **identifying** medical problems and initiating or modifying treatment;
2. **recording** smoking and alcohol consumption quantitatively;
3. **doing certain routine investigations if not done recently**
   (These are: Hb   all women
                 Sickle   all Afro-Caribbeans
                 CXR & ECG   all patients over 55 yrs.);
4. **doing other investigations (including the above) as clinically indicated** (This includes ECG and CXR from 45yrs if >15 cigarettes/day.); and
5. **ordering blood.**

Recommendations for blood transfusion requirements for particular operations are available on a printed card. Please indicate number of units ordered on the theatre list, as this enables the Theatre Receptionist to check (with a single phone call) that the lab. has received all requests.

Above all, contact us early if you are unsure about anything. The weekly anaesthetic rota is widely available; please use it to check which anaesthetist will be doing the list on each occasion.

The accuracy of the printed operating list is vital to safety, efficiency, and sanity: wrong ward or wrong order means badly timed premeds and lost porters, wrong operation means wrong instruments, wrong age can mean wrong-sized anaesthetic equipment: any changes **MUST get through to all the team**.

3 PCA—a better way to administer familiar drugs

In this chapter we will consider the basis for advocating PCA and for the choice of drug and dose regime.

POSTOPERATIVE HABITS

Modern advances in surgical treatment have been dependent on advances in anaesthesia. Putting it at its most basic, patients will only submit to, and survive, a limited range of procedures without pain relief and physiological support. Whilst everyone recognizes that pain usually persists after any form of trauma, most attention has naturally been directed to the operative period. For the majority of surgical operations the doctors have felt that they have discharged their duty adequately by writing a relatively standardized prescription for opiate drugs to be administered intramuscularly (IM) 'prn' (merely an abbreviation of the Latin for 'as the occasion requires'). In other words, analgesia is at the discretion of the nurse, who is left to look after the sufferer when the surgeon and the anaesthetist are busy with something else.

CHANGING TIMES

In recent years it has become more common for doctors and nurses to 'admit' to being patients and to write of their experiences. Almost universally, they express horrified disbelief at the amount of pain they endured and the inadequate methods available for its relief (Angell 1982; Foott 1978; *British Medical Journal* (editorial) 1976). Of course, it would hardly have been a story if they had felt all was satisfactory and no changes were needed; you may like to speculate on the contribution of the psychological factors discussed in detail in subsequent chapters, but, above all, remember that pain is what *the patient* feels: the carer can only imperfectly assess distress. The widespread introduction of recovery rooms and the trend towards shorter-acting anaesthetic agents have also made immediate postoperative pain far more obvious to anaesthetists, and these developments have helped, gradually, to overcome the very cautious attitude towards giving opiate drugs during this period.

WHY NOW?

The traditional regimes are certainly not completely incapable of giving good-quality pain relief (Jones and Harrop-Griffiths 1991). It seems likely that they worked better in the era when basic anaesthetic techniques left the patient with large depots of lipid-soluble agents such as ether and trichloroethylene, whose gradual elimination took many hours—the potentially most painful hours at that. These agents are significantly analgesic in their own right, and the dosage schemes that evolved took account of the additive effects of the residual anaesthetic and the administered opiate; importantly, the respiratory-depressant effects are also additive, and this factor will have had its influence on the quantities of opiate deemed safe on the basis of experience.

Shorter-acting opiates, less cumulative anaesthetic agents, and an increasing use of paralysing drugs instead of deep anaesthesia to prevent inconvenient reflex muscle activity have all given anaesthetists much better control. Many of the worries about airway maintenance, adequacy of respiration, and cerebral function that demanded recovery rooms are paradoxically restricted to a much shorter period with today's techniques. This increase in safety has been bought at the expense of greater susceptibility to and appreciation of the pain generated immediately after the trauma.

Control is desired by patients (people) as well as by anaesthetists—it is a feature of the rise of consumerism! Whether it be access to information or deciding where you live, recent trends are all towards rejection of those in authority in favour of the individual. When it comes to health, the doctor is the equivalent of authority, and needs to be an enabler rather than a despotic controller; viewed in this way, it is not surprising that PCA is a treatment of our time.

WHAT NEEDS CHANGING?

The worst features of the traditional 'prn' regime can be listed briefly:

● inflexibility—some patients need ten times more than others (Thomas *et al.* 1990);

● dependency—the nurse must be 'caught' and convinced of the need for pain relief; and

● delay—even then, the drug must be checked out with a second nurse, drawn up, injected into a muscle, and absorbed into the blood, and must finally diffuse to its site of action in the brain before any relief can occur.

The common result has been succinctly summed up—not enough and not often enough!

Box 6. *Drawbacks of the intramuscular regime*

Inflexibility
Dependency } Result: inadequacy
Delay

An Acute Pain Team can produce very marked improvements by encouraging pain assessment, information giving, and more liberal use of IM opiates (Gould *et al.* 1992). However, the intensity of activity required to achieve similar results would seem difficult to reproduce in most hospitals.

WHY PCA?

Patient-controlled analgesia deals with these deficiencies simply and effectively. The basic components of a PCA system are:

(a) a reservoir of the chosen opiate drug; connected to

(b) an intravenous cannula; and

(c) a control system that allows the patient to trigger release of a measured quantity of drug (the bolus dose), but will not respond to a subsequent patient demand within a preset time (the lockout period)(Fig. 3.1.).

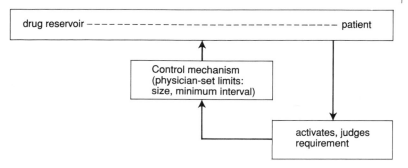

Fig. 3.1. Schematic representation of a PCA system.

The bolus dose is prescribed by a doctor, and is usually about one-tenth of the dose that would be prescribed IM. The lockout period is designed to give the bolus dose time to reveal its effects (both analgesic and depressant), so that the patient can safely seek further doses. Apart from the theoretical knowledge of how long it takes the drug to diffuse to its site of action, many small practical details also need to be taken into account in setting up the system and prescribing the lockout period; however, it is usually about 5–10 minutes. These facts give us a basis for a simplified comparison of the two systems using common prescriptions (Table 3.1): with the IM regime the patient is unlikely to obtain relief in less than an hour from feeling pain, but can get no more than this one dose of 20 mg in 4 hours; with PCA the patient is likely to get relief within five minutes, and could if necessary obtain 96 mg in 4 hours. Just as important as the greater amount available for a patient who needs a lot is the possibility for a very small total dosage: given that both our patients felt pain and 'requested' analgesia from the 'system', the patient on IM had to have 20 mg, but the one on PCA could have chosen to have only 2 mg in the 4-hour period. *Note*: Following a recent warning from the Committee on Safety of Medicines, papaveretum should not be prescribed for women of child-bearing potential.

Patients vary not only in their analgesic requirements but also in their susceptibility to side-effects: unpleasant (nausea, vomiting,

Table 3.1 Events in the pain-management cycle: 'IMI prn' and PCA compared, or FOUR HOURS IN THE POSTOPERATIVE EXPERIENCE OF TWO PATIENTS

PRESCRIPTION: papaveretum 20 mg IMI, 4-hrly prn	PRESCRIPTION: papaveretum 2 mg bolus, lockout 5 min. via PCA
Time: 21 00: PAIN Call nurse. Nurse accepts request. Finds chart, 2nd nurse, syringe, etc.; checks, gives injection, records.	Time: 21 00: PAIN Press button, bolus IV. Time: 21 05 RELIEF—if not, repeat every 5' until OK.
Time: 21 30 Drug absorbed. Time: 22 00 RELIEF (If you're lucky; if not, too bad!)	
Time: 23 30 PAIN RECURS: —sorry!	PAIN RECURS: Press button: RELIEF.
Time: 00 30 Getting worse: 'still an hour to go'.	
MAXIMUM in 4 hrs: 20 mg MINIMUM in 4 hrs: 20 mg	MAXIMUM in 4 hrs: 96 mg MINIMUM in 4 hrs: 2 mg

dizziness) and dangerous (respiratory depression, excessive sedation). So, the PCA system deals specifically with the three disadvantages cited above—inflexibility, dependency, and delay.

It is possible to get round some of the problems of the IM regime by increasing the nursing and medical time devoted to individual patients; staff who convince the patient that pain relief is possible and desirable, who respond promptly to individual requests, who assess the effects and alter the prescription will improve care accordingly. Their responses close the feedback loop between the patient's perception of pain and the treatment available somewhat more quickly. This type of responsiveness is appropriate for all patients in the recovery room and for selected patients who require closer supervision within the High-Dependency Unit (HDU) or Intensive Therapy Unit (ITU). But PCA shortens the pathway and increases the sensitivity, to achieve strikingly better results for all patients undergoing painful procedures.

WHY DO NEEDS VARY SO ENORMOUSLY?

Any clinical practitioner (nurse, doctor, or pharmacist) has expended time and effort learning about drug therapy for illness. Remarkably few disease states are described in our textbooks without a section on treatment that includes drugs. The nature of the drug, its presumed mechanism of action, its dangers, and its side-effects are always accompanied by a dose recommendation. For any given condition, the dose-range is usually quite narrow; and it is part of our normal thinking about drugs that most of the variability of effect is governed by differences in absorption or excretion, the route of administration, and such patient-related factors as age, sex, and weight; and that there is a target blood level which will be effective.

All these sources of variability may affect opiate drugs, of course; but there is a very fundamental difference when it comes to the concept of a target blood level. Part of the problem is the condition under treatment: there is such a wide range in the amount of stimulus, which is determined not only by the volume of damaged tissue but also by the sensitivity of different parts of the body. The action required of the analgesic drug has virtually nothing to do with modifying the abnormal process: it has to act on a distant organ stimulated by the process. Opiate drugs act on receptors in the brain which are specialized to react with compounds that are naturally present—the endogenous opioids. The complexity of the receptor systems and the controlling mechanisms for the production of the endogenous opioids are still in the process of being appreciated and understood. Several excellent reviews (Yaksh *et al.* 1988; Pleuvry 1991) demonstrate that at the moment the subject defies simplification. Fortunately, it is not difficult to grasp the idea that a patient with a lot of endogenous opioid may require very little additional analgesic to give pain relief, whereas one with very little will need a lot. This is sufficient for most of us to accept the reality of the differences that can be demonstrated daily in the recovery room. Two patients of the same weight, age, and sex may have, for example, a hernia repair performed by the same surgeon under identical anaesthesia, including the same modest amount of analgesic. One will awake and require to be convinced that the operation has been performed; the other will surface in obvious distress, and may require very large amounts of intravenous opiate (a total of 20 mg of morphine is not unusual) before comfort is achieved. Clearly, endogenous opioid production and receptor sensitivity are likely to be the pathways through which psychological factors such as anxiety have the marked effects that have been demonstrated on pain perception and opiate requirements; these factors are discussed further in Chapter 4.

Other factors that contribute to variability of requirements in postoperative patients include impairment of kidney or liver function, which may affect the excretion or metabolism of certain drugs, and hypovolaemia or hypoproteinaemia, which can affect the dilution volume or protein binding of drugs, thus altering the concentration of drug free to diffuse to the active site.

Since the reason for giving opiates is to get the patient as near to his or her chosen level of comfort as possible, it seems attractively simple to accept the impossibility of calculating the correct dose and merely set limits which allow the patient to achieve this end with safety. The target is comfort, rather than a single, universally correct blood level.

Box 7. Factors affecting the pain experience of different patients

● Amount of trauma = basic stimulus
● Personality—underlying susceptibility
● Present anxiety—increased susceptibility
● Metabolic and physiological disturbances

WILL A SINGLE PATIENT NEED VERY DIFFERENT DOSES AT DIFFERENT TIMES?

If individual patients commonly displayed the same sort of variability in their requirements over short periods of time as is displayed by the whole population, the safe and effective treatment of pain would be very difficult indeed by any method. As the ability of research workers to measure analgesic drug concentrations in the blood and to distinguish active metabolites has improved, clinical assessment has been supplemented by accurate data on blood levels and the concept of the minimum effective analgesic concentration (MEAC) has evolved (Austin *et al.* 1980*a*). It has been shown that not only do patients exhibit a relatively constant individual blood level at which analgesia is achieved, but that the difference between the blood levels at which no effect and full effect are perceived is remarkably small (Austin *et al.* 1980*a*). When first introduced PCA was principally used as a research tool, allowing patients to titrate themselves to their desired comfort level. This can be used to exclude observer bias in the comparison of different analgesic drugs or regimes; and, by allowing the patient to top-up the effects of a test substance with an established effective drug, many ethical problems are overcome. Research of this type has established that in the first 24–48 hours after painful surgery, individual patients demand drug at a remarkably constant rate (Hull and Sibbald 1981), indicating that there is indeed a target effective blood concentration, but that it can vary markedly (Austin *et al.* 1980*a*), contributing to the tenfold variation in consumption seen between individuals (Hull and Sibbald 1981).

Keeping in mind the idea that individual blood levels are important, Fig. 3.2 illustrates another way of comparing IM with PCA. Two patients need postoperative pain relief; they look pretty similar, so they have both been written up for the same analgesic regime, although in fact B needs nearly twice as much as A. Blood levels A1 and B1 represent the MEAC for each patient (the threshold for pain relief). Levels A2 and B2 are those at which disliked side-effects such as nausea occur (this occasionally is much closer to or is even lower than the MEAC). A3 represents the level at which dangerous side-effects are seen. At A3 patient A has significant respiratory depression.

On the IM regime (Fig. 3.2 (i)), the patients awake and complain of pain and, with minimum delay (for this is an efficient recovery room), each of them receives his or her injection. Blood levels rise, and after a further 10 minutes patient A feels thankfully comfortable; but not long after she feels a bit sick, and receives some metoclopramide. Some fifteen minutes later however, she becomes quite sleepy, and when supplementary oxygen is removed

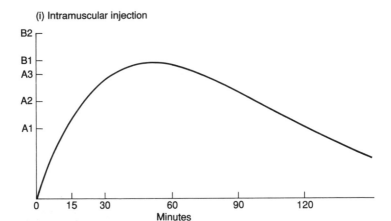

(i) Intramuscular injection

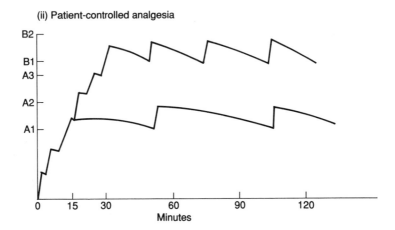

(ii) Patient-controlled analgesia

Fig. 3.2. Comparison of analgesic blood levels following IMI or PCA in two patients (A and B) with markedly different requirements.

Patient A needs only half as much analgesic as patient B. A1, B1 represent blood levels of analgesic which A and B respectively find to produce comfort. A2, B2 are the levels at which they notice side-effects (for example nausea or drowsiness). A3 is the level at which respiratory depression leads to a drop in oxygen saturation in patient A.

before handover to the ward nurse, her oxygen saturation falls and the oximeter (it is also a well-equipped recovery room) alarms. The oxygen is replaced and she is instructed to breathe deeply, the nurse is sent back to the ward: 'We'll keep her a bit longer.' As the blood level falls, the patient once again reaches the happy state of being comfortable and not oversedated, and can therefore return to the ward. However, only two hours after her injection, her blood level falls below the MEAC, and she starts to be distressed again; but her request for analgesia brings forth the response: 'I'm sorry, you're not due for any more for another two hours.'

Patient B simply never gets to an appropriate blood level: from some points of view he is quite safe; but what if the tachycardia engendered by his pain compromises myocardial blood-flow?

With PCA (Fig. 3.2 (ii)), the two patients have been connected to the system on entry to the recovery room, so that as soon as they complain of pain they are instructed to press the button, and encouraged to repeat this each time the lockout period expires and they are still not comfortable. Patient A achieves comfort soon after the third press—little more than ten minutes later, although B takes nearly half an hour. Neither experiences side-effects, and each soon returns to the ward and settles into his or her individual characteristic demand rate—A triggers a bolus approximately every 50 minutes, and B every 25 minutes. The time-concentration profile of an IM injection is not the full explanation for the inferiority of such regimes. Intravenous bolus doses will produce consistent changes unless very marked changes in blood volume occur. IM injections however, exhibit serious variations in absorption within and between individuals (Austin *et al.* 1980*b*): maximum blood levels vary nearly threefold, and may occur any time between 20 and 100 minutes after injection; thus even if a given dose proves satisfactory on one occasion there is no guarantee that the same dose repeated later will have the same effect.

FACTORS THAT MATTER LESS THAN WE TEND TO THINK

Given similar operations, there is virtually no evidence for body weight as a significant factor in analgesic requirements in the adult population, although men need more drug than women and younger people need more than older ones. In one study (Burns *et al*. 1989) which looked at these factors the males used almost one and a half times as much morphine in twenty-four hours as the females, and sixty-year-olds used less than half as much as thirty-year-olds. These generalizations, although significant, are of little predictive help, since the individual consumptions ranged from 5 mg to 165 mg—a 33-fold difference. Weight was not correlated with consumption, and dosage ranged from about 0.075 mg/kg to 3.4 mg/kg—an even greater difference. The dose requirements in children and adolescents have received little research attention; but it is clear that the adult findings cannot be simply transferred. Neonates are sensitive to opiates, and the very large difference in body weight must be a factor. The age-dependent metabolic differences that determine the increased sensitivity in old age are mirrored at the other end of life (Lloyd-Thomas 1990), with immaturity of breakdown pathways. Metabolic differences will produce differences in both the height and persistence of the blood level for similar drug doses, and therefore the variation in drug consumption with age is greater than the variation in effective drug concentration (Kaiko 1980).

Box 8. Factors leading to significant but minor changes in opiate requirement

• Age
• Sex
• Circulatory state
• Time of day

THE BASIS FOR CHOICE OF DRUG

The factors to be considered include length of action, effects on mood and cognition, cumulation of metabolites, and gastro-intestinal side-effects. Speed of onset via the intravenous route is sufficiently rapid for all available opiates to be satisfactory from this point of view. The length of action should be such that once a level of comfort has been achieved the patient does not have to repeat demands too frequently; at the other end of the scale, the possibility of acute changes in the patient's condition make very long action a disadvantage, and, in addition, patients seem to appreciate a degree of change in the analgesic level. Well-established drugs, such as morphine, diamorphine, papaveretum, and pethidine, have the advantage of familiarity within the postoperative scene. Papaveretum (originally a mixture of morphine, codeine, papaverine, and noscapine) has recently come under a cloud as a result of the possibility that noscapine could be teratogenic. It has however a very long history of apparently satisfactory use, and a noscapine-free formulation (Omnopon Roche) has now been introduced.

Newer drugs, developed specifically to have a shorter duration of action and less additional effects, such as fentanyl and alfentanil, have been used mainly as part of balanced anaesthetic techniques. They have also been used for PCA, which can be seen in this context as an attempt to extend intravenous anaesthetic techniques into the postoperative period. Almost all published studies have claimed good results for PCA whether or not they compare it with other regimes, whatever the drugs used, so, one might say that it matters little which drugs are chosen. We feel, however, that there are some grounds for distinguishing between what is available. There is little doubt that clinically significant differences will emerge from the many studies currently being undertaken, and cumulative clinical experience as the technique becomes more widely used. Neither do we rule out the possibility that new drugs will be introduced with more suitable profiles in terms of cumulation, nausea, and mood change, although respiratory depression seems to be inextricably linked to analgesia.

LESS SUITABLE DRUGS

Certain characteristics seem to us to make pethidine, alfentanil, and fentanyl less suitable than others. Pethidine metabolizes to nor-pethidine, which accumulates during long-term usage, and has been implicated in the causation of dysphoria and convulsions (Smith and Elwood 1988; Mitchell *et al.* 1991; Pryle *et al.* 1992). The action of alfentanil is so brief that patients find it very difficult to achieve stable blood levels, and thus effective analgesia, even with additional infusions (Currie *et al.* 1990). Fentanyl has been used effectively (Rowbotham *et al.* 1989*a*); but its relative lack of sedative or mood-modifying effects seem to make it less liked by patients than the morphine family, and in addition its relatively short duration of action seems to require the patient to make demands with a frequency that could be tiresome. In one study (Welchew and Breen 1991) demands were made on average every 12 minutes during the first twenty-four hours, and the highest user apparently made demands almost every four minutes! There also seem good common-sense reasons for rejecting other possibilities such as methadone (too long-acting), pentazocine (limited analgesia, plus the risk of hallucinations), buprenorphine (both long-acting and difficult to antagonize), and meptazinol and nalbuphine (too emetic).

MORE SUITABLE DRUGS

Diamorphine has given very satisfactory results in a District General Hospital service (Notcutt and Morgan 1990), and it has been suggested that its higher lipid-solubility might give it advantages over morphine in terms of speed of onset both of analgesic effect and possible accompanying respiratory depression (allowing immediate recognition) after intravenous injection. Although studies have not substantiated these advantages (Annan *et al.* 1988; Morrison *et al.* 1991) the important point is that both drugs revealed their effects extremely quickly (within one to two minutes). Similarly, rather little difference has been demonstrated with regard to nausea, sedation, or sense of well-being (Robinson *et al.* 1991), despite widely held clinical opinions of diamorphine's advantages.

Many studies, particularly those from the Flinders Medical Centre in Australia, have testified to the good results obtained with morphine. We are concerned, however, at the results of a study (Aitkenhead and Robinson 1989) on patients undergoing large-bowel resection where the effects of morphine and pethidine on anastomotic failure rates were compared, morphine being associated with a significantly higher rate. In addition, there has been a recent report of acute pancreatitis apparently precipitated by spasm of the sphincter of Oddi consequent on the use of a morphine infusion supplemented by PCA (Mills and Goddard 1991). The effects of morphine on bowel motility and smooth-muscle tone are well known, and it is unlikely that diamorphine differs in this respect;

further research is clearly needed to determine whether this effect should be taken into account, and whether spasmolytic therapy is indicated. It is therefore possible that papaveretum may have some advantage in this type of case, as the papaverine component acts as a peripheral spasmolytic. It is difficult to assess the importance of this factor; but PCA, by lowering the total amount of drug required to produce adequate analgesia, should minimize the effects on the gastrointestinal tract whichever drug is chosen. Although we still favour papaveretum where suitable, morphine (its principal active constituent) is clearly safe and effective, and has been successfully used in a District General Hospital Acute Pain Service (Wheatley *et al.* 1991). The effects of the older opiates on mood combine a degree of sedation with euphoria, and are usually liked by patients.

Box 9. Features of drugs whose use for PCA has been described

Drug:	alfentanil fentanyl	pethidine	morphine	diamorphine	papaveretum
Length of action	too short	OK	OK	OK	OK
Cumulative breakdown products	OK	toxic	OK	OK	OK
Smooth muscle spasm	?	reduced	increased	increased	reduced
Mood	little effect	sedation± euphoria	sedation± euphoria	sedation± euphoria	sedation± euphoria

---

SETTING THE LIMITS—BOLUS DOSE AND LOCKOUT TIME

We have been at pains to stress the very wide range of doses needed by different patients to achieve comfort. However, in the regime of PCA that we would advocate we recommend relatively small bolus doses (0.5 mg of diamorphine, 1 mg of morphine, or 2 mg of papaveretum) to minimize unpleasant side-effects in susceptible patients. But in view of the wide range of doses required by different patients there is one very obvious potential drawback to this policy, particularly in the initial postoperative situation:

a technique that relies on small intravenous doses can maintain an effective blood concentration well but is not a good way of reaching it from scratch, especially if the patient happens to need a high concentration.

The use of moderate doses of analgesic will allow a proportion of patients to recover consciousness within the range of comfort. But for those whose distress shows that they are well below the MEAC it is particularly important that a low-dose PCA regime should be coupled with and preceded by a period of reasonably bold intravenous titration to good analgesia by the anaesthetist within the safe confines of the recovery room. Thus, for example, Patient B in Fig. 3.2 could have been brought to a comfortable level in a shorter time by receiving IV doses of 2–2¹/2 times the bolus dose chosen. It is very likely that patients with high requirements at this stage will remain high users, and might benefit from a higher bolus dose right from the start. None the less, on balance we still recommend the relatively low-dose scheme outlined above since it will minimize unpleasant side-effects and has the advantage of allowing a simple initial protocol. Adjusting the regime for optimum results is discussed in Chapter 11. Using a higher bolus dose as standard (double those suggested) will give good pain relief and may be considered more practical if early review is not possible.

The lockout time can be kept to the minimum required to ensure that significant effects from one dose (analgesia and respiratory depression or sedation) are appreciated before a further dose demand is accepted. As discussed above, this could be as short as 2–3 minutes. However, it is important to be sure that no significant part of the lockout period is taken up by delays in the drug's actually reaching the patient's circulation. This possibility is discussed in more detail in other chapters, but, briefly, could be caused by a slow pump infusion rate (unlikely with modern equipment unless deliberately specified); by a large volume to be delivered; or by deadspace needing to be traversed by the bolus (additional connections or even a very-large-bore cannula combined with a slow drip-rate, where the PCA is attached as a side-arm to an IV infusion). So long as these conditions are carefully avoided, preferably by using a dedicated cannula, there is no evidence that increasing the lockout interval beyond five minutes confers any extra safety with the drugs recommended; but very large studies would be needed to detect such effects on what has so far proved to be an exceptionally trouble-free technique.

WHY NOT INFUSIONS INSTEAD OF, OR IN ADDITION TO, BOLUS DOSES?

Part of the effectiveness and acceptability of PCA has been attributed to reducing the wide fluctuations in blood level caused by infrequent, large, intramuscular injections. There is an attractive apparent logic to the suggestion that providing at least part of the opiate continuously as an infusion (termed a background infusion) could reduce the fluctuations further, with even better results. Indeed, sophisticated systems have been devised that compute the rate of bolus demand dosage over any one hour, and deliver half this amount as an infusion during the next hour (Hull 1985). Evidence is accumulating, however, that even very low-level background infusions increase the amount of drug used without improving results (Owen *et al.* 1989; Parker *et al.* 1989). There is evidence that, within the relatively fixed characteristic individual dose rate, there is a distinct diurnal variation (Graves *et al.* 1983; Burns et al. 1989) that is not obvious when operation time (rather than a particular time of day) is used as the reference start-time. Allied to this, it seems that patients like to experience a degree of fluctuation in the level of pain relief: it may increase the sense of control that contributes so much to many patients' enthusiasm for the system; or they may seek occasional mild sedation at a time they judge to be appropriate, maximizing the chance of dropping off into natural sleep. In addition, the incidence both of reductions in respiratory rate to levels that may indicate significant depression, and of upper respiratory tract obstruction are very much higher when background infusions are used (Notcutt and Morgan 1990; Wheatley *et al.* 1991). Doctor-prescribed opiate infusions can provide very effective pain relief, but only at the expense of a significant level of dangerous sedative and respiratory-depressant effects (Catling *et al.* 1980). This is not at all unexpected given the very wide range of dose requirements for pain relief. One study has reported that patient-controlled infusions, with carefully set conditions, gave superior pain relief to conventional PCA in cancer patients with acute pain (Hill *et al.* 1991). In Chapter 14 we discuss the probable reasons for these particular findings, which seem at odds with the main body of evidence. We feel that there is a consensus developing amongst experienced workers that infusions are neither safe nor useful for the majority of situations.

WILL PATIENTS PUSH THE BUTTON OFTEN ENOUGH?

It might be thought that keeping the bolus dose very small would be another method of reducing fluctuations in blood levels, and thus perhaps side-effects. A lockout period of five minutes allows patients to make twelve effective demands per hour (assuming that the time taken to deliver the dose is negligible); and certainly, at the start of therapy and with appropriate encouragement, patients can be persuaded to keep repeating demands until they are comfortable. Similarly they will accept the need to seek extra doses close together in anticipation of some painful event, such as drain removal or getting out of bed. However, few patients have the tenacity or desire to make demands more frequently than every 20 minutes throughout the postoperative period, and will usually reject the equipment if the bolus dose is not adjusted appropriately. Unexpected results from some studies can become easier to understand if the demand rate is calculated from the consumption and bolus size data. Unless unpleasant nausea or dizziness is caused by the size of bolus needed, we suggest that patients would prefer only to have to make a demand about once an hour.

WILL IT WORK FOR EVERYONE?

Most workers who have used PCA for research purposes report that a proportion of patients, perhaps as many as 5 per cent, simply will not activate the PCA machine, although they appear to be in sufficient pain to require analgesia. It seems that they are frightened of the idea of being in charge of a 'high-tec' machine. Ever since the introduction of PCA, great stress has been laid on the need to explain the system to the patient preoperatively. Some anaesthetists feel it is necessary to demonstrate the actual equipment to them. As we discuss in Chapters 4 and 5, we regard the provision of appropriate information on all aspects of treatment to patients as extremely important, particularly on the grounds of reducing fear of the unknown as a stress-provoking stimulus. The crux of the problem is the nature of the appropriate information and the way it is given to the patient. It is clearly possible to give frightening information or to give the right sort of information in a frightening way. In addition there are a few patients (though we feel probably very few) who really cannot bear to know anything in advance. In a study involving the administration of several psychological questionnaires preoperatively, a necessary part of the design precluded giving information about the way postoperative pain relief would be provided (Thomas *et al.* 1990). The patients were asked by recovery nurses on awakening whether they needed anything for pain. Those that were randomized to receive PCA were given the handset to press when necessary, and encouragement was continued on the postoperative ward. None failed to use the system; the only problem encountered was rejection of the system after a few hours by one patient because of inadequate pain relief: almost certainly the bolus dose was inappropriately low for her needs. This finding illustrates how difficult it may be to be sure that information is appropriate. We certainly do not reject the general value of information, and it seems likely that some of our patients would have been happier or used the system better with prior explanation.

In addition, there are some patients who are so sensitive to the emetic effects of opiates that they will reject any regime involving them. Other methods of pain relief need to be explored for this type of patient.

4 Social and psychological aspects of postoperative pain experience

1. FACTORS TO BE TAKEN INTO ACCOUNT

Background

There are a number of reasons for seeking the provision of effective control of postoperative pain. Severe pain causes misery which affects the quality of life, and its control is therefore desirable on humanitarian grounds. Apart from suffering, pain is likely to exacerbate a number of postoperative complications that impede recovery. Immobility, induced by fear that any movement may cause pain, increases the likelihood of complications such as deep vein thrombosis, chest infections, and pressure sores. The report on *Pain after surgery* (Royal College of Surgeons and College of Anaesthetists 1990) notes that these complications are less likely in pain-free patients, and that musculoskeletal function also recovers more rapidly.

The amount of pain following surgery is, on average, predictable from measurable and objective surgical factors; however, there are other factors affecting the experience of pain irrespective of the method used for its relief. These include cultural background, age, sex, individual personality, and other psychological variables.

Cultural and ethnic factors

The reactions of a wide range of cultural and ethnic groups have been studied under a variety of conditions, in both clinical and laboratory settings. It is now clear that the experience of pain cannot be fully explained without reference to cultural and ethnic differences, although, sadly, very few of these studies have been conducted in the postoperative situation.

Whilst cultural differences undoubtedly exist, they appear to be differences in expressiveness rather than in the sensory experience (Melzack and Wall 1988). Cultural norms regarding behaviour when in pain—when to and where to express pain—are learnt at an early age (Peck 1986; Thomas and Rose 1991). People of Latin origin are typically more expressive, and are inclined to dramatize pain expression with elaborate vocalization and posturing (Zborowski 1952; Lipton and Marbach 1984; Migliore 1989). The stoical Scandinavian, on the other hand, is more likely to become withdrawn and uncommunicative (Chapman 1984). Black people have been found to complain of more pain than whites (Woodrow *et al.* 1972), although more recent research seems to contradict this, and has found black people to tolerate pain better than whites, and whites better than Asians (Thomas and Rose 1991). This pattern was also found in the postoperative situation. For example, Miller and Shuter (1984) found that white postoperative patients reported more pain and, in describing pain, they used words of more variety and greater intensity than did black patients.

Differences in analgesic consumption can be seen as a measure of pain tolerance, and can also be attributed to culture. Streltzer and Wade (1981) conducted a study to assess the doses of analgesics given after surgery in relation to cultural background. They found that Caucasians and Hawaiians received significantly more analgesia than Chinese, Japanese, or Filipino patients. Accurate assessment of pain and response with appropriate relief depend on precise interpretation and validation of the patients' communications. Although these researchers suggested that their result was due to nurse-patient interaction they did not make any reference to the ethnic origin of the nurses, and this may well be important.

Cultural background of staff

The cultural background of the nurses may be very relevant, since this is likely to interact with that of the patient and influence both pain experience and analgesic consumption. Nurses share common beliefs that certain operations, injuries, and illnesses are more painful than others, and that some conditions cause greater psychological distress than others. Research indicates that nurses also share the stereotypical belief that patients from particular ethnic or religious backgrounds differ markedly in the degree to which they suffer. In a cross-cultural study of nurses' perceptions of pain and suffering (involving 1400 nurses of various ethnic groups from 13 countries), Davitz and Davitz (1981) utilized 60 vignettes, each describing a patient and his/her medical condition. The nurses were asked to rate the amount of physical pain and psychological distress associated with each condition. The results showed that nurses from different countries differed in their inferences of both dimensions: the results are sufficiently striking to warrant summary. They illustrate not only that nurses, in the course of caring for patients, have formed views of racial characteristics involved in pain experience, but also that the cultural background of the nurses themselves influenced these generalizations.

Nurses believed that Jewish and Hispanic/Spanish patients suffered most on both dimensions, whilst Oriental and Anglo-Saxon/Germanic patients suffered least; other groups fell between these extremes. Nurses of North European culture inferred the least physical suffering, whilst those from African and Southern European backgrounds inferred high levels of suffering. Nurses from Asian countries showed a wide range of national differences in their inferences of both psychological distress and physical pain: the Koreans inferred the most of both, with the Japanese next. Whereas Taiwanese and Nepalese accorded the lowest scores for psychological distress, with Thai nurses higher, the latter inferred the least physical pain, with Taiwanese, Nepalese, and Japanese inferring increasing amounts. Puerto Ricans assessed psychological distress to be high but physical pain low, whilst English, American, and Belgian nurses expressed the lowest ratings for physical pain of all the cultural groups. There is reason to believe that these views are not confined to nursing staff, but are also held by medical staff (Hartog and Hartog 1983). These diverse results illustrate the difficulty of generalizing about pain on the basis of race.

In British hospitals, surgical patients come from a variety of cultures, and are cared for by a multicultural staff. If a nurse or doctor infers less pain than the patient reports, the patient is labelled a complainer, and evokes irritation and anger in the staff. Davitz and Davitz (1985) reported that British nurses working in American hospitals found it difficult to cope with patients from non-European backgrounds. They found American, South American, and Puerto Rican patients particularly demanding and more emotionally expressive. Culturally-based approaches to the management of postoperative pain must be tempered with certain precautions since, if used in a negative way, they may not be significantly different from prejudice. A caring approach is essential, and will tend to overcome any cultural mis-step (Hartog and Hartog 1983). With very few exceptions (Thomas and Rose 1991) the bulk of the research concerned with ethnic differences has been conducted by white researchers. The element of trust which considers whether blacks and other ethnic minority groups like relating to white authority figures and vice versa requires investigation. Some patients might feel able to disclose more to a particular nurse or doctor because they consider him or her to be more sympathetic as a result of cultural background. For example, an Afro-Caribbean patient might feel more able to report pain to a nurse from the same culture because she/he gives him/her 'permission' to express pain that a nurse from another culture would not. These cultural differences may significantly contribute to pain experience and analgesic consumption in the postoperative period, and require further investigation in hospitals serving and staffed by a diversity of people.

Gender differences

The evidence concerning the influence of gender on pain is conflicting: Glynn *et al.* (1976) found that pain scores amongst chronic pain patients were higher for females than males, whilst Khun *et al.* (1990) found no such difference amongst postoperative patients. Both Miller and Shuter (1984) and Nayman (1979) found that less pain was experienced by males, although only in the former study did the results reach statistical significance.

Using the amount of analgesia consumed as an indirect measure of pain experience adds a layer of complexity. Bond (1981) found that male patients on a radiotherapy ward received less analgesia than females, and similarly Taenzer *et al.* (1986) found that, in surgical patients, females required significantly more analgesics than males; however, Burns *et al.* (1989), using PCA to allow patients to adjust their medication, found that males consumed significantly more than females. Neither Nayman (1979) nor Streltzer and Wade (1981) could find significant differences in amounts of medication given to males and females postoperatively.

Age

The effect of age on pain experience is also not simple. In an attempt to determine age-related variation in analgesia and pain experience among postoperative patients, Kaiko (1980) conducted a study of 946 surgical patients ranging from 18 to 89 years of age. Enhanced analgesia was associated with age: 50 per cent of the oldest groups experiencing an average of 5 hours of pain relief compared to 3 hours for the youngest group. Kaiko concluded that the duration of analgesia rather than peak effect is responsible for age-related differences and that this may be the result of a decline in the function of organs responsible for drug breakdown and elimination. These findings are supported by the studies of Belville *et al.* (1971); Berkowitz *et al.* (1975); Taenzer *et al.* (1986); and Mather and Mackie (1983).

However the picture is further complicated by the differences in the amount of pain reported by different age-groups. On the one hand, Miller and Shuter (1984) found that patients over 40 years reported more pain than younger ones, yet Khun *et al.* (1990) on the other hand found no differences. Overall there seems to be good evidence that age has an important effect only on the optimal dosing interval for analgesics.

Personality of the patient

Psychometric techniques provide the means of measuring different aspects of personality such as neuroticism, extraversion, and anxiety-proneness. Personality can affect the pain sensation or the expression of pain (Dodson 1985), and it is not easy to separate these two factors. Bond (1973), studying chronic pain patients, found that high neuroticism scores accompanied high pain scores, and high extraversion scores were associated with increased pain complaints. Sternbach (1978) has argued that neuroticism and introversion would naturally inhibit pain complaints. However, while the information on personality gained from the study of chronic pain patients is of value, caution should be exercised in generalizing from this. In the acute postoperative situation, pain may serve to reduce the intense feeling of loss (Bond 1984); for instance, it may substitute for the loss of a part of the body, as after hysterectomy or limb amputation. The significance of the pain is therefore an important variable which may interact with the personality factors to be described.

Extraversion

Extraversion reflects the patient's sociability. Several studies (Dalrymple and Parbrook 1976; Boyle and Parbrook 1977; Taenzer *et al.*

1986) have failed to find any relationship between extraversion scores and postoperative pain, assessed in various ways. The last-quoted study (of 40 cholecystectomy patients) did find, however, that extraversion score was significantly predictive of the amount of analgesic used. This probably reflects an association with willingness to seek medication and the ability to convince nurses of need.

Neuroticism

Neuroticism refers to a person's emotional stability, and is considered by Eysenck (1967) to be involved in measures of trait anxiety (see below); this has been supported by Loo (1979). In an early study, Cronin *et al.* (1973) were unable to demonstrate any relationship between neuroticism and either pain experience or amount of medication used; later work, however, has shown significant associations. In their study of 190 patients undergoing upper abdominal surgery, Boyle and Parbrook (1977) found that neuroticism correlated positively and significantly with the amount of pain experienced by both men and women. They also found that postoperative impairment of lung function and the incidence of chest infections correlated with high preoperative neuroticism scores. Lim and colleagues (1983), studying 30 similar patients, observed a correlation between preoperative neuroticism scores and postoperative morphine requirements which accounted for 80 per cent of the variation.

In a study of 52 patients, designed to predict the dose of methadone required after surgery, Gourlay *et al.* (1982) found that neuroticism and social conformity scores accounted for the largest proportion of the variation in requirement. Similar results, with positive correlations between neuroticism and both reported pain and analgesic usage, have been found by Taenzer *et al.* (1986) and Thomas *et al.* (1990).

Anxiety

The association between anxiety and pain is well known, and anxiety is by far the most commonly reported and researched preoperative emotion. Indeed Sternbach (1968) asserts that 'all that is necessary for maximizing pain responses is that anxiety responses also be great'. Despite thorough exploration of this relationship, the source of the anxiety has been disputed. Understanding has been aided by the distinction made between 'state anxiety'—

a transitory emotional condition that varies in intensity, fluctuates over time, and is associated with particular circumstances—and 'trait anxiety'—a personality disposition that predisposes people to become anxious (i.e. to demonstrate state anxiety) in stressful situations (Spielberger *et al*. 1973). Spielberger's State/Trait Anxiety Inventory has been used in most of the studies referred to below, to clarify the association between anxiety and postoperative pain.

State anxiety

People awaiting surgery become extremely anxious: about the anaesthetic, postoperative pain, and the possibility of death (Carnevali 1966). Admission to hospital is in itself stressful, and impending surgery heightens this anxiety (Wilson-Barnett 1979). Not surprisingly, state anxiety has been found to increase through the whole period immediately before hospitalization, and it is noteworthy that the highest levels occur just after operation (Johnston 1980). Various studies of preoperative state anxiety and its relation to postoperative pain experience and/or analgesic requirements have consistently demonstrated significant correlations (Scott *et al*. 1983; Lim *et al*. 1983; Thomas *et al*. 1990). Postoperative state anxiety and pain are also highly correlated (Seers 1987).

Earlier studies, whose relevance to current conditions cannot be certain, have attempted to tease out complex relations between preoperative anxiety and outcome. The work of Janis (1958), suggesting a curvilinear relationship between preoperative fear and postoperative emotional disturbance, led to the proposition that moderate preoperative anxiety is associated with a better outcome. Janis's explanation was that patients with low preoperative anxiety do not engage in cognitive preparation and consequently become angry and resentful when confronted with the reality of postoperative discomfort. On the other hand, the highly anxious patient has unrealistic fears, and remains fearful after surgery. Subsequent research has only weakly supported this hypothesis. Whilst Auerbach (1973) found that surgical patients with moderate anxiety levels expressed more positive feelings about hospitalization than those with either low or high levels, Johnston and Carpenter (1980) found that low anxiety was associated with a slower rate of recovery than moderate anxiety. The latter researchers concluded that, on the whole, preoperative anxiety was a poor predictor of recovery.

Trait anxiety

The stability of trait anxiety scores during the perioperative period has been demonstrated by Auerbach (1973) and Spielberger *et al.* (1973), justifying the distinction between it and the fluctuating state anxiety. Trait anxiety has been shown to correlate with postoperative pain by Martinez-Urrutia (1975), Taenzer *et al.* (1986), and Thomas *et al.* (1990). In an interesting study of 67 renal donor and recipient patients, Chapman and Cox (1977) found that it was predictive of pain, state anxiety, and depression in recipients, but not donors. The authors argued that the perioperative situational anxiety was affected by the meaning attached by the patient to the surgery: thus the recipients were affected by the knowledge that their new kidney might be rejected. This particular study is difficult to evaluate because of the number of factors operating at the same time, since patients receiving a donated kidney usually have a long history of chronic disease and its associated problems. Chronic pain patients have a higher incidence of depression, which can also intensify pain (Fordyce 1976). They may also have developed 'learned helplessness' as a coping strategy (see below). It seems possible, therefore, that chronic renal patients may consider the pain associated with their condition to be inescapable, and this preset schema could have interacted with the surgical situation.

Other workers, using different measures of anxiety such as Taylor's (1953) manifest anxiety scale (Johnson *et al.* 1971) and the modified S-R inventory of anxiousness (Wolfer and Davis 1970 and Hayward 1975), have in the main failed to predict postoperative pain, the amount of analgesic consumed, or the length of hospital stay; however, Hayward's (1975) study did report a positive correlation between trait anxiety and length of stay. Such discrepant findings may be attributable to inadequate measures either of anxiety or of recovery (Mathews and Ridgeway 1981). Nevertheless, it does appear that anxiety as a personality characteristic can play an important role in postoperative pain experience, and also in the likelihood of developing complications.

Helplessness/loss of control

Loss of personal control over the environment is a great source of stress, and significantly contributes to the anxiety experienced by surgical patients. The most basic human rights, involving mobility, privacy, and even control over bodily functions, are often taken over by hospital staff. After surgery, the patient is frequently helpless, attached to tubes, unable to move, and totally dependent on others. Responses to pain are likely to be greater under these circumstances. Patient-controlled analgesia makes a significant contribution to the reduction of suffering simply by giving the patient a degree of control, in addition to the contribution of its impact on the pain itself.

Summary

It seems that there are many psychological factors which can influence postoperative pain. Ethnic and cultural factors, age, and gender are significant elements of the setting in which the patient undergoes surgery; but the patient's personality profile, anxiety level, and degree of control are the most important and interactive determinants of pain experience. The relationship between the concepts of control, anxiety, and postoperative pain will therefore be considered in detail in the next section.

2. INTERACTIONS BETWEEN CONTROL, ANXIETY, AND POSTOPERATIVE PAIN

Exerting control over one's environment can affect both safety and comfort, and there is evidence that lack of control is aversive and anxiety-provoking (Peck 1986; Chapman and Cox 1977). Most individuals find the prospect of impending surgery stressful. The probability of experiencing pain, the loss of immediate personal control, and the potential loss of the ability to resume normal activities are all sources of stress (Auerbach 1979). It has already been shown that anxiety is an important determinant of postoperative pain; and many theorists have emphasized a complex interaction of physiological mechanisms and the psychological state of helplessness in accounting for anxiety (Mandler 1972; Lazarus 1966). It seems plausible that uncontrollability may be a factor common to both anxiety and pain, and many studies (human and animal) support the link between perceived control, anxiety, and painful or aversive events (Mandler and Watson 1966; Henry and Stephens 1977; Katz and Wykes 1985).

Definition of control

Thompson (1981) defined control as the belief that one has at one's disposal a response that can influence the aversiveness of an event. This definition is particularly useful because it recognizes that, for it to be effective, control does not have to be exercised (potential control), and that it does not even have to be real as long as it is believed to exist (perceived control). Thompson has identified four types of control: informational, cognitive, retrospective, and behavioural.

Informational control

The content of a message and its delivery can take many forms: it can be a warning signal that precedes a painful stimulus, and therefore gives information about the timing of the event; or it can be a message about some characteristics of the situation or stimulus. The provision of adequate information to a person about to undergo surgery reduces the uncertainty, and thus the distress.

Cognitive control

Cognitive control is the belief that one has a cognitive strategy available which can affect the aversive event. A wide range of cognitive strategies has been used in pain research, but, in essence, they can be classified as avoidant or non-avoidant. Avoidant strategies lead one to ignore, distract, or dissociate oneself from the event, whilst non-avoidant strategies cause one to focus on the event through heightened sensitivity and attempt to control physiological or cognitive reactions.

Retrospective control

The assumption here is that reinterpretation of the causes of a past painful event will alter its current implications; it has no great relevance to the management of postoperative pain. Indeed, all of these first three types of control, whilst of some value, are essentially passive.

Behavioural control

This refers to any behavioural response that can actively influence the perception of pain, making it less probable or less intense, or changing its duration or timing. Simple examples include keeping the injured area still and reducing anxiety by controlled breathing exercises. Patient-controlled analgesia (Sechzer 1968) is clearly a sophisticated form of behavioural response to perceived or anticipated pain.

Research evidence on the importance of the different types of control for surgical patients

Informational control

Information given preoperatively allows patients to interpret their surroundings and circumstances and to anticipate postoperative events (Boore 1978). Correctly managed, this can engender a feeling of control and reduce helplessness (Monat, Averill, and Lazarus 1972), thus reducing anxiety (Mandler 1972). Procedural information, offered by the anaesthetist preoperatively, has been found to reduce both the need for postoperative analgesics and the length of hospital stay (Egbert *et al.* 1964). Vernon and Bigelow (1974) found that informed patients were more satisfied and knowledgeable, and more likely to anticipate pain, but less likely to deny thoughts of the operation when compared with an uninformed group. Similarly, Hayward (1975) compared patients given detailed procedural information with those given a similar amount of simple attention, and found that anxiety and reported pain were both reduced.

A few studies have examined the way in which preoperative procedural information alters physiological indicators of stress: Boore (1978) demonstrated a reduction in postoperative infection rate and in corticosteroid excretion—but the experimental group were also taught breathing, leg, and abdominal exercises, which can have both behavioural and physiological effects in addition (Thompson 1981).

Although information reduces anxiety, it is more effective if it focuses upon what the patient is likely to experience (sensory information) rather than the objective nature of the procedure. Johnson (1983) considers that this type of information provides the patient with an imaginary map. Effective sensory information is chronologically structured, includes details of common sensations, and is confined to the patient's vocabulary. Many studies have confirmed that terms that are very familiar to staff are not understood by most patients (Cosper 1967; Byrne and Edeani 1983). 'Blown out', 'sticking', 'pounding', and 'gurgling' are examples of the sort of sensory words that are understood by patients, but somehow do not seem to be used much by staff. Johnson has carried out a number of influential studies that have distinguished between procedural and sensory information. In an early study (1973) of gastrointestinal endoscopy patients, sensory information was more effective in reducing restlessness and overt signs of tension, whilst in cholecystectomy patients (1978) there was a reduction in postoperative stay and in the time before patients first ventured from home. However, no differences were found in terms of pain, mood, or initial mobilization.

Whilst the distinctions are interesting, the best effects seem to be achieved by combining sensory and procedural information. Ridgeway and Mathews (1982) compared this strategy to an equivalent amount of simple attention, and found reductions in preoperative anxiety, in annoyance related to waking up at night in hospital, and in days of pain after discharge. Anderson (1987), studying patients undergoing major cardiac surgery, confirmed reduction in preoperative anxiety and found additional benefits in terms of reduced negative emotions and improved nurse ratings of physical and psychological recovery, as well as a reduction in the levels of postoperative hypertension. Similarly, Davis (1984) found that a combined sensory, procedural, and behavioural information package reduced the severity of postoperative pain in patients undergoing upper abdominal surgery. Zeimer (1983), however, found the addition of sensory information added nothing to the benefits of procedural information in a group of abdominal surgical patients. Postoperative delirium has been a common complication in some studies of patients undergoing open heart surgery and of elderly patients undergoing various types of surgery; it has therefore been given special attention. Many risk factors have been identified: these include advanced age, magnitude of physiological disturbance, preoperative anxiety, and personality factors (Rogers and Reich 1986). In this difficult area, some of the investigative efforts have inadvertently altered the responses by providing preoperative information interventions. For example, Kornfield *et al.* (1974) unexpectedly discovered that a single preoperative interview with a psychiatrist reduced the incidence of delirium after surgery by 50 per cent. This study also revealed that patients with the personality traits of dominance, aggressiveness, and self-assuredness were at greater risk of experiencing delirium. In another study, Owens and Hutlemeyer (1982) simply informed patients of the possibility of experiencing the unusual perceptual disturbance associated with delirium. Although there was no statistical decrease in incidence, patients thus prepared reported feeling more comfortable and in control than the unprepared control group. This study shows another facet of the importance of the sensory component of the information given to patients preoperatively.

The interaction between information and coping style

Whilst the general trend of the work reviewed so far appears to indicate that knowing what will occur gives the patient a degree of control and helps to reduce anxiety related to the unknown, not all patients benefit from detailed information. Indeed, it appears that such information can have the opposite effect: Langer *et al.* (1975) reported that simple information had the effect of magnifying pain by causing patients to focus on the discomforting aspects of the experience they were about to undergo, and Kanfer and Goldfoot (1966) also reported that specific sensory information reduced pain tolerance, possibly by sensitizing subjects to the pain they were about to experience.

'Coping style' refers to the kind of strategies that people adopt in threatening circumstances, and to their desire for information in uncontrollable situations. In general, people either seek out information about the threat—a 'monitoring' or 'vigilant' coping style—or they distract themselves from such information—a 'denying' or 'blunting' coping style. It seems that the patient's coping style is an important moderator of how detailed information will be utilized. Andrew (1970) found that preoperative information could be detrimental to individuals who used denial as a coping strategy, and Miller (1980, 1987) showed that preoperative information was most effective when it took account of the patient's strategy for either attending to ('monitoring'), or ignoring ('blunting') the threatening situation. Patients with a high-information preference have been shown to do better after surgery if given combined sensory and procedural information (Auerbach *et al.* 1983; Miller and Mangan 1983).

The perceived locus of control may also interact with information. Individuals with an internal locus of control typically believe that their health is under their own control, whereas those with an external locus of control suppose that luck, faith, or powerful others (such as health-care professionals) have control over their health. Research evidence suggests that 'internals' may benefit more than 'externals' from detailed information. Auerbach *et al.* (1976) studied oral surgical patients and found that improved recovery followed specific information for 'internals', whereas 'externals' did better with general information presented prior to surgery.

Uncertainty over how to use information, even when it has been presented in accordance with personality style, may reduce benefit (Clum *et al.* 1979), and the provision of information within a context that includes guidance on how to use it will enhance effectiveness (Rogers and Reich 1986). The provision of information in suitable booklet form has been shown to reduce pain and to speed recovery when compared with the provision of nothing but oral information (Klos *et al.* 1980). It seems likely that preoperative fear interferes with attentional processing, and a booklet allows the patient the opportunity to take in information at a slower and/or more varied pace.

Cognitive control

Changing the perception of helplessness is central to the therapeutic endeavour, and the belief that one has a cognitive strategy is valuable in the surgical situation. Attempts to give the patient control will not be entirely successful unless the patient actually feels in control. A number of studies have looked at the effectiveness of reinterpretation as a cognitive control strategy that can be taught to patients preoperatively. Reinterpretation requires the patient to focus on the more positive, beneficial aspects of the procedure, such as 'postoperative pain will be relieved by painkillers and it does not last long'. Langer *et al.* (1975) found such a strategy effective in reducing preoperative anxiety, analgesic requirement, and length of stay after major surgery. Ridgeway and Mathews (1982) taught reinterpretation strategy to hysterectomy patients, and found that they had better sleep patterns, required less oral and injected analgesic medication, and reported less pain. This group also had a reduction in the number of symptoms, and were more self-caring at home three weeks after surgery. Kendall *et al.* (1979) found that a combination of reinterpretation, calming self-talk, and relaxation taught to patients about to undergo cardiac catheterization had favourable effects on adjustment and anxiety.

In another combined cognitive strategy intervention, Wells *et al.* (1986) exposed hysterectomy and cholecystectomy patients to a combination of self-monitoring, distraction, self-statements, and relaxation, and showed lower levels of pre- and postoperative anxiety, less postoperative pain, better nurse ratings of adjustment, and marginally lower use of analgesics and shorter hospital stay compared to an untreated control group. In a more selective study Pickett and Clum (1982), on the other hand, found that distraction was more effective than relaxation in reducing pain and anxiety after cholecystectomy.

Hypnotherapy has also been used as a form of cognitive control. Bonilla *et al.* (1961) studied patients undergoing knee surgery; the preoperative hypnosis group were given posthypnotic suggestions: that they would not fear surgery, that they would be aware of pain but not be bothered by it, and that they would be able to exercise the knee immediately after surgery. By comparison with controls, the group required less analgesics and had a shorter average rehabilitation time. Although similar results were obtained by Kolouch (1964) in general surgical patients, Surnam *et al.* (1974), using autohypnosis together with a therapeutic interview, were unable to show an effect on analgesics used or on postoperative complications. There was, however, a reduction in length of stay. These mixed findings highlight the fact that patients differ in their acceptance of hypnosis and have a variable capacity to respond to it for either pain control or other purposes. Kolouch (1964) identified that the usefulness of hypnosis was limited both by the magnitude of surgery and by unspecified personality problems.

There is thus some evidence that cognitive control, either alone or as an adjunct to other strategies, can be successful in reducing pain and speeding recovery. More recent studies have begun to take account of broad differences in pre-existing emotional states and coping style. This approach can allow psychological interventions to achieve more clinically significant contributions to surgical outcome.

Behavioural control

Behavioural control is the most active form of control available to the surgical patient, and the desire for control increases when patients have more information about the situation they are about to confront (Schorr and Rodin 1984). Cromwell *et al.* (1977) found that the most deleterious effects upon recovery occurred when patients had a great deal of information and no actual control by participation in care. Averill (1973) identified two types of behavioural control: regulated admission (control over the circumstances surrounding pain experience, such as when it occurs) and stimulus-modification (ability to modify the actual level of pain in some way). Patient-controlled analgesia is a clear example of the latter; but both types of control are highly relevant to surgical patients. Most postoperative pain is intensified by movement of the affected area, and, particularly after the first twelve hours or so, patients may not be in pain at rest. They can therefore decide precisely when they will have pain and, to some extent, how severe it will be. The decisions on when, how, and how much they will move or breathe deeply enhances the sense of control, but may have serious effects on mobilization, and thus on complications such as thrombosis and chest infections.

Several investigations have examined the impact of progressive muscular relaxation as a means of the regulated-admission type of behavioural control strategy for surgical patients. Aiken and Henrichs (1971) incorporated relaxation into an intervention which also gave the opportunity for open-heart patients to talk about their fears, and showed improvements in anaesthesia time, bypass time, and degree of hypothermia. Similarly, Wilson (1981) found that with relaxation there was a reduction in pain medication, better recovery, increased reports of strength and energy, and a quicker discharge; these effects were greater for low-fear than for high-fear patients. Teaching abdominal surgery patients a relaxation technique for getting out of bed (Flagherty and Fitzpatrick 1978) or specific coughing techniques (Lindeman and Van Aernam 1971) were found to reduce pain and improve vital capacity respectively. However, Smith (1974) failed to show any significant effects on pain control or length of stay from a progressive muscular-relaxation technique.

Patient-controlled analgesia as a behavioural control

The behavioural-control element of PCA is an example of stimulus-modification. Other features of the control aspect of PCA include the ability of the patient to retain privacy. This is important because the common methods of pain relief require the patient publicly to acknowledge pain, and, for various cultural and personality reasons, some patients feel that pain is a private experience, and will therefore suffer in silence rather than request analgesia from a nurse. Few studies have as yet been carried out on the interaction between personality and the need for active control in the postoperative situation. Johnson *et al.* (1988) measured locus of control in 40 hysterectomy patients in an attempt to determine whether it could be used to predict the effectiveness of PCA. They found that patients with an external locus of control experienced more pain, and inferred that this group of patients did not like taking control. Coping style has also been used to predict the need for active control via PCA. For example, Wilson and Bennett (1984) measured coping style preoperatively, and assessed factors such as avoidance, independence, emotional stability, and aggressiveness. They found that patients with high levels of independence and emotional control used less analgesic medication. High levels of independence were also associated with lower pain scores.

The 'monitoring' style of coping is also an important predictor of the effectiveness of PCA. Thomas (1991) preoperatively assessed coping style in 164 surgical patients, and found that 'monitors' experienced less pain than 'blunters'. These results are consistent with the informational-control literature. Since a monitoring style reflects a desire for control, this result suggests that 'blunters' (those with low desire for control) experienced more pain because they did not like to exercise the control they were given with PCA. Clearly, this area deserves further exploration.

Why does control reduce pain?

Several hypotheses have been advanced to explain the finding that the various forms of control can be demonstrated to reduce pain in some situations. All have an implicit assumption that stress, anxiety, and pain are integrally related.

Predictability hypotheses

The safety-signal theory (Seligman *et al.* 1971) suggests that control is beneficial because it allows the individual to predict when the painful stimulus will occur: if a signal reliably predicts danger, then the absence of the signal reliably predicts safety and relaxation. An individual with an actual behavioural control has more safety-signals, and in the postoperative situation this can account for part of the effectiveness of systematic relaxation and PCA.

Berlyne's (1960) information-seeking theory similarly seeks to account for control intervention findings in terms of predictability. These theories cannot adequately account for those patients who do not gain beneficial effects from information, nor for the apparent willingness of individuals to tolerate more intense levels of pain when a behavioural control is present. Separating the features of controllability and predictability has shown that the former has effects over and above the latter (Geer and Maisel 1972). Since these theories are present-time-orientated, focusing on the advantage of control in decreasing anticipatory anxiety, they do not account for the long-term positive effects that have also been found for preoperative control strategies. Johnson's (1973) incongruency hypothesis seeks to explain the effects of sensory information in the postoperative situation in terms of reduced incongruency between expected and experienced sensations. It suggests that severe pain occurs because of a discrepancy between what is expected and what is experienced, and that reducing this will also reduce attendant anxiety. This hypothesis is therefore more useful in explaining the longer-term effects, and support for this view comes from Epstein (1973), who proposed that accurate information facilitates habituation. However, the theory does not adequately explain the reduction in preoperative anxiety, nor the effects of interaction between information and personality style.

The Minimax hypothesis

Other theorists have focused on controllability as a message about outcomes. Miller's (1979) Minimax theory proposes that patients with control responses can minimize maximum future danger. Specifically, such patients know that pain will not become so intense that they cannot cope with it because they can invoke relief from a stable, internal source: their own response. Although developed to explain the effects of behavioural control, the theory can also be applied to cognitive and informational control, since these also engender strong beliefs that pain will not exceed bearable limits, thus accounting for reduction in preoperative anxiety. The Minimax theory also predicts that, in some situations, individuals will prefer to have no control because control is in the hands of another person (for example, a skilled professional) who is better placed to minimize harm and pain. This versatile theory has been extended (Miller 1981) by the 'Blunting' hypothesis, which addresses the changes in information-processing, and appears to integrate the contradictory literature on informational control in the postoperative situation. Emphasis is placed on the ways in which cognitive processing of information by individuals may reduce stress reactions. Stress will remain high in the uncontrollable pre- and postoperative situations if patients are alert for, and thus sensitized to, the negative aspects of the surgery. Miller suggests that high levels of information generally increase stress and anxiety, because they force the individual into the psychological presence of an unavoidable danger. Lower levels of information, on the other hand, decrease anxiety and ultimately pain, because patients are able to absent themselves from cues about the operation. This makes it easier to engage in blunting strategies such as distraction; for some people this will effectively reduce anxiety.

In accounting for studies which have achieved positive effects from high-level, detailed information strategies, Miller has suggested that accurate expectations have promoted less surprise and therefore less overt behavioural signs of pain. According to Miller, the interaction between coping style and the impact of information means that 'monitors' (high-information-preference patients) fare better with detailed information, whilst 'blunters' (low-information-preference patients) cope better with stress by distraction. Monitoring is seen as the most stressful behavioural style, and is associated with greater subjective and behavioural distress in the perioperative period (Miller and Mangan 1983). The blunting hypothesis can also account for the success of reinterpretation techniques which cause the patient to focus exclusively on positive aspects of surgery, and for the success of distraction as a coping strategy.

Thompson (1981) states that a common theme running through all the literature on control is the meaning of the event for the individual. Thus she concludes that controllability does not influence painful events; rather it is the meaning of the event which is the crucial factor. Early studies of pain noted that the meaning of an injury or its consequences dramatically affected the amount of pain felt (Beecher 1956; Melzack and Wall 1965). Arntz and Schmidt (1989) suggested that the inferred harmfulness of the pain is a central issue; control over pain causes changes in its meaning, and hence in the way it is experienced. They further propose that pain can be controlled if it is perceived as harmless, and therefore has a different significance for the patient. On the other hand, pain that cannot be controlled is perceived as harmful, and has a negative effect on the individual simply as a consequence of its inescapability.

The endurable-unendurable aspect of the meaning of pain is an important dimension captured by the assurance within the Minimax hypothesis that pain will not be beyond the limits of endurance; it can be seen as analogous to the harmless-harmful dichotomy in the perception of pain explored by Arntz and Schmidt (1989), and helps to explain many of the effects of informational, cognitive, and behavioural control interventions in the postoperative patient. It is useful in explaining the finding that PCA patients use less medication and yet report less pain, on the basis that PCA gives the patient both behavioural control and decisional control. The provision of PCA adds another important aspect to the endurable-unendurable dimension by giving the patient the right to decide what is or is not endurable. The fact that some patients use less medication in this situation suggests that the knowledge of one's own control increases endurance.

However, although the meaning of the situation is an important concept in the experience of pain, it is but one link in a complex chain. In considering pain in the surgical context, Johnson's idea that sensory informational control reduces incongruency has an important role. However, Miller's (1979) idea that control minimizes maximum pain, and her blunting hypothesis, which states that attention to pain increases it whilst distraction decreases it, is also consistent with the findings. These two theories appear to account for most of the positive effects of informational, cognitive, and behavioural control, whilst taking account of the interaction between personality style and control.

Conclusions

It is useful to summarize these wide-ranging findings. Hospitalization and subsequent surgery are events over which surgical patients often have no control. This stress is compounded by acute postoperative pain. If individuals believe that they have no control over a painful event, their anxiety level increases, and itself contributes to increased pain perception. Control does not have to be exercised to be effective, neither does it have to be real for it to have positive effects. In the postoperative period both perceived (cognitive and informational) and actual (behavioural) control manipulations have shown their ability to reduce anxiety and pain levels and to promote a speedy and uncomplicated recovery. There is an interaction between personality style and control such that some patients prefer control, whilst others reject it. This may lead some patients to reject PCA or to use it ineffectively; and therefore studies are required to increase our understanding of the application of appropriate information and cognitive strategies in conjunction with PCA in different personality types.

5 Information and PCA

PREOPERATIVE INFORMATION

The importance of information

Impending surgery with its special features is a major source of stress for the surgical patient, but evidence also exists which suggests that admission to hospital is in itself very stressful (Wilson-Barnett 1979). Factors identified as important include isolation, loss of autonomy, and separation from spouse or other key family members. The provision of information to the surgical patient is important because it reduces uncertainty and promotes accurate expectation of surgical experience, and therefore provides some element of control in what is otherwise perceived as an uncontrollable situation.

How to give information

Establishing a starting point is vital. The patient needs to know who you are and what your level of responsibility and area of expertise is: name badges should be large enough to read without peering. It is advisable to remember that 'house surgeon' may sound strictly analogous to 'tree surgeon'. You need to know how much patients already understand and what their expectations are.

Although the majority of patients benefit from information because it reduces surprise, there are some individuals who prefer to know very little because they 'like to take things as they come'. Therefore, before information is proffered to the surgical patient, a rough assessment of his or her desire for information should be undertaken. In its simplest form this involves asking the patients straightforward questions about the amount of detail they would like to have regarding the surgical procedure and possible experiences. It can be important to distinguish between different areas: they may like to know what will happen whilst they are awake, but not whilst they are under anaesthesia. French (1979), in a study of 312 surgical patients, found that 16 per cent said that knowledge was upsetting and that they preferred to avoid the 'sordid details'. This is a clear indication of the sensitivity required during the information-giving, and it takes little imagination to appreciate the difficulties of research in this area. There are also potential difficulties if long-term matters such as the reasons for and seriousness and effects of the surgical procedure have not been dealt with properly within the out-patient and GP consultations. These concerns can block uptake of quite simple explanations. Previous experience will naturally affect the patients' views and needs. It is possible to save a lot of time by checking the notes, especially the correspondence between GPs and specialists. Patients gain confidence if you demonstrate a good grasp of their previous histories, and in these circumstances they will more easily relate good and bad experiences.

Box 10. Assessing informational needs

● ?level of existing knowledge
● ?desire for detail
● ?previous experiences

In the bewildering context of hospital admission, patients are greatly helped if explanations of procedures are given with strict regard for the chronological sequence of events (Wilson-Barnett 1988). Keeping to the right order allows the patient to build a framework within which the entire episode can be fitted, and is a help to containing the emotional impact. Explanations should focus primarily on what patients will see, feel, and hear; the language used **must** be that familiar to them. Technical terms not only add to the stress: their incomprehensibility is likely to lead to patients' 'switching off' to subsequent information, however well presented. Research has shown that medical terminology, even for example 'premedication', is not easily understood by patients (Byrne and Edeani 1983). It is better to describe what will happen in simple, direct words: 'I think it is a good idea if you have a tablet of a tranquillizer just to settle you down during the last hour or two before coming up to the operating department; the nurse will give it to you here with a little water. Is that OK?—you don't have to have it.' If the patient responds with 'Is that the premed?' nothing has been lost; on the contrary, the fact that they can feel clever will help their confidence!

Unfamiliarity with medical matters and lack of general education must not be equated to lack of intelligence or any particular level of need for information or ability to take it in. Research has shown that general practitioners volunteered fewer explanations to patients of lower social class, believing that they understood less and therefore required less (Pendleton and Bochner 1980). Of all social groupings, this group have probably the greatest need for information to be offered to them, because they tend not to ask many questions pertaining to their care (Pendleton and Bochner 1980). Disregard of the need for a bit more effort in ensuring comprehension will add another layer to the feeling that their health is the responsibility of the clever professionals, and that their own choices (for example on life-style and smoking) are of marginal relevance.

These considerations also apply when providing information for patients of different cultural groups. If British patients find the terminology used by medical staff incomprehensible, what chances are there for patients from ethnic minorities whose grasp of the English language is limited? All efforts should be made to ensure that sufficient information is provided for these groups, and this includes the use of interpreters and translations of written information. The giving of information should be a sharing experience, so that patients have the opportunity to discuss worries, both general and particular. In trying to elicit concerns from the patient, open-ended questions are very useful, because they allow the patient to talk more freely, revealing attitudes about illness: 'How are you feeling about your operation?', rather than 'Are you worried about your operation?'—the latter approach is likely to provoke a straight 'yes' or 'no', neither of them necessarily true, and both certainly not particularly helpful. Although the greatest preoperative fears of surgical patients are the severity of pain and other discomfort (Wilson-Barnett 1988), they have other worries which may be perceived by nursing and medical staff as unimportant. For example, many patients become very worried at the prospect of being dependent on nurses for things they would normally do for themselves, particularly matters involving privacy (French 1979). Such matters need to be explored whenever they are identified. As well as advising patients about strategies that will be useful in dealing with particular problems, it is important to involve patients and ascertain what they think might be good ways of solving problems. Interventions will be more successful if they accord with patients' cultural norms, values, and belief systems.

The essence of an effective approach is a calm, unhurried manner, and the time required for this must be acknowledged. It has been suggested that twenty minutes is an appropriate length of time (Wilson-Barnett 1988). However, each member of the professional team will have his or her own needs and time-scale. Too much information of marginal relevance to the particular patient will be an unhelpful distraction; direct contact should be carefully directed to the individual.

Box 11. Verbal information

● Tailor to individual
● Keep time-sequence
● Encourage feedback

Written information must perforce be more general, but is nevertheless extremely valuable both as a reinforcement of verbal communication and as a source of facts about areas that may not have been raised. Relatively young staff may find it difficult to discuss sexual matters, for instance, with older persons, or may be unable to conceive the relevance of doing so. Patients should also be encouraged to write down any worries and problems they could not remember at the time of interview, so that these can be dealt with at another time: the patient bearing a written list should not be regarded with a sinking heart, but rather as an intelligent contributor to efficient health-care collaboration. Regrettably, we must include a reminder that a significant proportion of the adult population is functionally illiterate, and that some are amazingly ingenious at concealing this fact; take care that they do not feel more disadvantaged than is necessary by the failure of our education system—Einstein had great difficulty learning to read. The use of diagrams should be maximized: they are an efficient means of communication for all ages, and can reduce the need for translations.

Lay organizations such as the major health charities are often most successful in the field of written communication. They too have access to the best professional factual advice, but are often better at judging appropriate styles of layout and language. Their involvement can clearly contribute economies of scale by covering those areas that are not hospital- or person-specific. Specialist units need to develop a hierarchy of leaflets, so that a mix-and-match selection can be made for each patient. As far as possible, tatty photocopies of undifferentiated typescript should be replaced by attractive, well laid out printed leaflets. Including a request that they should be returned so that another patient can benefit has a surprising effect on the perceived value of the content, as well as of the paper!

Box 12. Written information

- Make it attractive
- Use appropriate language
- Use diagrams
- Grade levels of detail
- Consider translations

In general, staff should concentrate on giving information related to their own area of knowledge. Wherever possible, a suitable (usually brief) note of what has been conveyed should be made in the notes. This becomes particularly important where matters of prognosis or complications are tackled, and is vital on those occasions when one is trapped into dealing with some matter not strictly within one's own remit, but where failure to make a response would seriously damage a patient's confidence in the care team.

GIVING INFORMATION ABOUT PCA

Although patients can use PCA devices effectively after surgery despite not being told about it beforehand (Thomas *et al.* 1990), most patients will appreciate being introduced to PCA systems preoperatively, and will adapt more rapidly to using them appropriately as a result. Patients need to be educated about the basic principles of PCA (as set out later in this book) and encouraged to use it to control their pain after surgery. Ideally they should be shown the system that they will use and have the activation mechanism demonstrated. After this they should be allowed to try 'button-pressing' under supervision.

Clearly, limitations on the number of machines available mean that this ideal will rarely be achieved with the computerized pumps. It is, however, possible to purchase spare handsets for demonstration purposes. The disposable system can be refilled with water for demonstration purposes; it is most important that the distal Luer connection is cut off to ensure that it can in no circumstances be connected to an IV line.

Whoever provides the initial information about PCA, the nurse on the ward has a crucial responsibility for allaying patients' fears and highlighting the safety aspects of PCA. A common question posed by patients is 'What if I give myself too much pain killer?' Unless this anxiety is properly dealt with suboptimal use is very likely. The nurse should emphasize that the anaesthetist will take account of their individual reactions during anaesthesia in choosing the dose, and that the predetermined lockout interval and regular nurse assessments ensure that overdosage is virtually impossible. Current practice in UK does not demand that every possible complication must be drawn to the attention of patients—only those that have a measurable incidence. For this we must be thankful, since untold anxiety can be generated preoperatively. Nevertheless, some patients will enquire very persistently about such matters. A judgement has to be made about how to handle such people. Usually we would favour absolute honesty: this is made somewhat easier by the absence of fatal accidents involving PCA in UK.

If possible, close relatives should also be given an explanation of PCA, because they may be alarmed to find the patient attached to technically sophisticated machinery without prior explanation. It has to be said, however, that many view such equipment with extraordinary equanimity, and it is equally important that they should be expressly forbidden to activate the equipment on behalf of the patient. Compliance is best achieved if they are made to understand that safety depends on patients themselves controlling the release of the drug. Although there are a few circumstances (such as small children undergoing painful surgery) where this rule must be broken, it should only be broken in the most carefully controlled and supervised circumstances.

A most effective way of reducing fear of the unknown is talking to someone with firsthand experience—someone for whom this 'unknown' has become a familiar and positive event. So introducing the patient preoperatively to someone recovering from surgery who has used the PCA system can be a most valuable way of providing reassurance. Nurses can enlist patients' help in this way, although care has to be taken that misconceptions are not passed on. Experience with the obstetric analgesia service has taught experienced practitioners a certain wariness both of enthusiasts and of detractors who base their views on isolated individual experiences. This avenue is probably best kept as a back-up for the pathologically anxious patient who has initially rejected the idea, and for whom PCA is paradoxically most beneficial.

It is as well to remember at all time that most patients like to please, and that this desire often manifests itself as a good impersonation of comprehension even when in reality little has been absorbed. In addition, patients (and professionals) often think they understand something when they have actually got hold of the wrong end of the stick. It is wise to seek feedback wherever possible, and to have protocols of observation and regime-review that will pick up misunderstandings. A recent report illustrates this well (Johnson and Daugherty 1992): a patient received an exceptionally full explanation of a PCA pump, including the fact that a green light would come on at the end of the lockout period to indicate that a further dose of analgesic could be demanded if desired. On review she was found to be pain-free but unusually drowsy, and it transpired that she thought that she needed to press the button every time the green light came on—further explanation led to a marked drop in consumption, with no diminution in the quality of pain control.

The information sheet that we use for patients is reproduced in the Appendix to this chapter. Copies are kept on the wards, and one in a plastic folder is attached to each machine—partly as a way of reminding staff that information may be 'better late than never'. Such sheets need to take account of different types of equipment.

Box 13. Information for patients about PCA

- Promote basic understanding
- Show equipment if possible
- Identify anxieties
- Inform relatives
- ? arrange talk with another patient
- Check adequacy of understanding

INFORMATION FOR STAFF

Promoting a hospital-wide appreciation and understanding of PCA seems to be one of the most difficult things to achieve. Even enthusiasts get weary of coaxing people to re-examine their concepts of safety in relation to opiates. Commitment from a majority of the anaesthetic department has to be a minimum starting-point; progress from then on requires a campaign to involve nursing staff in Recovery and on the wards, to convince Management of the soundness of the case and that it justifies the costs in equipment and staff time, and to guide successive cohorts of new staff—anaesthetic, surgical, and nursing. Clearly the more people who can be drawn into an information cascade the better. The most effective person will be a nurse specifically appointed to co-ordinate all aspects of the service. If sufficient equipment and time can be provided early, things go much more smoothly, because familiarity is rapidly gained and there can be confidence in offering the technique to patients preoperatively. If very few pumps are available staff will not expend time getting involved, in view of the possibility that it will be wasted; worse, there is a strong negative effect if you may have to apologize to the patient that the improved method of analgesia cannot be used after all.

Each group of staff need to be clear about their own responsibilities, as well as having a general understanding of the system and the service arrangements. The Anaesthetic Department policy has to cover setting up the equipment, suitable regimes, and documentation. Ward staff need to know what they are expected to do and who to contact when in doubt. Information sheets covering these aspects are included in the Appendix to this chapter;

however, they need frequent updating as different problems and practices evolve.

The concept of patient-controlled analgesia is relatively new for patients and staff alike, and it is important that those who have experience and expertise are encouraged to share this with others. As use of the technique increases, opportunities for such exchanges will also increase. In addition to patients returning to Lewisham Hospital for further surgery requesting (beseeching) the provision of PCA, we have already had a few requests on the basis of the experiences of friends and relatives.

APPENDIX: PATIENT-CONTROLLED ANALGESIA IN LEWISHAM HOSPITAL, MAY 1992

Anaesthetic department policy

Introduction

Experience to date with PCA suggests that it is a safe and effective system for postoperative pain relief, acceptable to patients and ward nursing staff. This policy is intended to highlight key points and inform staff not familiar with PCA without seeking to be restrictive or to remove responsibility from individuals prescribing and caring for individual patients.

Patient information: Patients can have the system explained to them at the preoperative visit; some have advocated actually showing them the machine. At Lewisham we have found it satisfactory to set up the system in Recovery without any prior introduction: the nurses there explain to and encourage the patient as they come round, and the ward nurses continue the process on transfer. Patient information sheets and feedback forms are available in the Anaesthetic Department. A copy of the patient information sheet has been sent to each ward, so that it should be available at the preop visit; in addition a copy is attached to each pump, and can be read to patients or given to them or their relatives to look at as soon as they feel able.

Prescribing: Use 'as required' section of chart. Write bolus dose in 'dose' box, 'via PCA' in 'route' box, lockout interval in 'max.

freq.' box. In 'additional information' record syringe contents thus: '120 mg of papaveretum in 60 ml saline = 2 mg/ml'. An 'average' woman, prescribed a bolus of 2 mg omnopon with a lockout of 5 min will use about 50 mg in 24 hours post-hysterectomy; there is a considerable range, and it is worth avoiding the syringe emptying during the hours of darkness! **Prescribe appropriate antiemetics.** If patients are at all nauseated in Recovery I suggest an IV bolus of 10 mg of metoclopramide as the most effective first step—whether or not they have had any recently. Nausea is the most common reason for distress/ dissatisfaction with PCA.

Oxygen: consider the need for additional oxygen in the light of increasing evidence of hypoxaemia, especially at night, in postoperative patients receiving opiates by ANY route.

Monitoring: Write appropriate monitoring requirements: respiratory rate is a poor indicator of respiratory depression, and good general observation is much more important; patients should not be put in siderooms.

Setting up: Draw the drug into the correct type of syringe (60 ml Plastipak for the Grasebys), dilute with saline or water, check the calculation of the dilution with the nurse issuing the drug, complete and attach the syringe label, and attach and prime the line.

Set pump to 'reprogram' with key (if unplugged it will run on the battery). Insert syringe, making sure that plunger is correctly held by drive and that barrel flange is securely in its slot. Program pump according to menu prompts. Plug into mains near the patient, and attach line either to dedicated cannula or to side-arm of non-return connector, which is then inserted into the main IV line: minimize deadspace by putting connector directly on to cannula; drip goes on to straight channel so that one-way valve prevents opiate backing up into drip if cannula is occluded. Turn key to ON and press 'run' or 'start'. Give the handpiece to the patient and instruct appropriately (Palliators and Graseby 3300s need **two presses** within one second, Graseby PCAS only needs a single press).

Transfer to ward: Do NOT turn key, as this will abolish the program. All that needs to be done is to unplug from the mains;

the pump will run on the battery until plugged in again on the ward. The Recovery nurse will ensure that instructions are noted and that the ward nurse understands the machine; she will also record the transfer in the PCA diary. Each pump has attached a copy of the patient information sheet and the information sheet for ward staff. On the ward, the pump can be stopped at any time, though this should rarely be necessary. The key (which is needed to open the syringe cover when refilling is required and to allow adjustments to the program) is kept on the recovery room controlled-drug key-ring, and, in the case of the Graseby PCAS pumps, must be borrowed from (and returned to) there. Each resident anaesthetist carries a key for the new Graseby 3300 pumps as well as the one that is kept in Recovery.

ONLY ANAESTHETISTS MAY ADJUST THE PROGRAM OR REPLACE SYRINGES.

We hope soon to reinstitute the evening round, when the duty pharmacist checks progress and alerts the duty anaesthetist to the need for either of these things. I am happy to be rung at any time about any problem (Home phone or Aircall via switchboard).

Advantages of the new Graseby 3300 pumps

Sensors ensure that syringe is correctly located in drive mechanism. They have been programmed to eliminate some options (e.g. background infusion, total dose limits) which are unnecessary for routine use. Programming is thus very simple: you only have to enter drug concentration, bolus dose, and lockout interval. The pump will only beep in response to a successful demand—this can be helpful to patients.

Margaret Heath, Consultant Anaesthetist

Ward staff information sheet

Introduction

Experience to date with PCA suggests that it is a safe and effective system for postoperative pain relief, acceptable to patients and ward nursing staff. Provision of PCA and supervision of the service is the responsibility of the Anaesthetic Department, whose policy document is available. This information sheet is intended to highlight key points and give some information to staff not familiar with PCA.

Principle

The PCA pump contains a syringe of dilute opiate, and is programmed to allow the patient to self-administer a very small dose intravenously when the handset button is pressed twice within one second (the two Graseby PCAS pumps only require one press to activate).

Thereafter, a 'lockout' period operates, so that another dose cannot be given without the full effects of the first being obvious. The advantage is that the effects are felt very quickly (in about three minutes) and that the very wide range of individual needs can be coped with: the usual IM regime means that most patients get delayed and inadequate analgesia, and a few get more than is good for them. There is also a tremendous psychological benefit to most patients from being in control of their own medication.

Patient information

Patients can have the system explained to them at the preoperative visit; some have advocated actually showing them the machine, but, unless this is done sensitively, some patients may reject the whole 'high-tech' idea. Patient information sheets are available (see pp. 70 and 71) and a copy is attached to the machine which you can either read to the patient or give to him or her to read when appropriate—make sure it gets reattached. At Lewisham we have found it satisfactory to set up the system in Recovery without any prior introduction: the nurses there explain the method and encourage patients as they come round, and ask the ward nurses to continue the process on transfer.

Prescribing

The anaesthetist will have written the prescription in the 'as required' section of the chart and set up the pump in Recovery. Antiemetics will also have been written up.

Transfer to ward

All that is needed on return to the ward is to plug in the mains lead to a wall socket and switch it on there; the pump will have been running on the battery during transfer and the program will have been kept. The equipment appears to be very safe and reliable but accidents can still happen—therefore,

PATIENTS ON PCA MUST NOT BE PUT IN A SIDE-ROOM

and should be easily visible at all times. Patients may need frequent doses to maintain comfort, and need to be encouraged to get themselves comfortable; they will not overdose themselves, because they will become too sleepy to operate the handset first. The patient's friends and relatives must be forbidden to operate the handset; very occasionally, patients may need help, particularly if they are arthritic. Help must only be given to a patient who asks for it. **Patients are the only people who really know how much pain they are in.** Nausea is the most common side-effect, so please ensure that antiemetics are given up to the maximum prescribed. If the symptom persists it may be necessary to adjust the size of the bolus dose and increase antiemetics. It should very rarely be necessary to discontinue PCA. Inadequate pain relief can result from too small a bolus dose or too long a lockout period—contact the duty anaesthetist (or me) if you think this is the case. Obviously, drip problems should be eliminated. If the PCA is attached to the sidearm of the main drip it is very important (a) that the drip is running at a reasonable speed and (b) that the arrangement of the one-way valve/cannula is not altered in any way. The pump will alarm if the cannula is occluded; but it is still important to check for tissueing, as in some circumstances this will not be detected.

The pump display will show how many doses the patient has taken, so it is possible to estimate when the syringe is likely to run out—please try to spot the patient with high requirements, so that the syringe can be replaced at a convenient time, possibly with reprogramming to a larger bolus dose.

ONLY ANAESTHETISTS MAY ADJUST THE PROGRAM OR REPLACE SYRINGES.

We hope soon to reinstitute the evening round when the duty pharmacist checks progress and alerts the duty anaesthetist to the need for either of these things. I am happy to be rung at any time about any problem (Home phone or Aircall via switchboard). I will give tutorials to any group of eight or more who can organize themselves to be free at a suitable time.

Alarm signals

Press the 'alarm' button to stop the noise. The pump display will tell you what the problem is; if you cannot correct it ring the prescribing anaesthetist in theatre (if the list is still going on) or the duty anaesthetic SHO. If neither is available, Recovery nurses will be pleased to give advice.

Length of treatment

We would like patients to have PCA for as long as they feel they need it. They should not get the impression that they ought to give it up as soon as possible—good analgesia speeds recovery (there is an average of two days reduction in hospital stay after hysterectomy for patients on PCA compared with IM prn). Even if the drip is no longer needed the PCA pump can be left attached directly to the cannula. When PCA is finally discontinued, record the total amount of drug used on the prescription chart opposite the PCA prescription, and return the pump and all attachments to Recovery.

Anaesthetic Department,
Lewisham Hospital

PATIENT-CONTROLLED ANALGESIA:

PATIENT INFORMATION SHEET

YOUR COMFORT AFTER THE OPERATION

May 1992

YOUR COMFORT AFTER THE OPERATION

During your operation your anaesthetist will ensure that you feel no pain by using anaesthetic and pain-relieving drugs. As the effects of these wear off you are likely to feel some pain; the degree of discomfort varies a lot—a very few lucky people have little or no pain, but after most major surgery some pain relief is required. Research here has shown that allowing patients to control their own pain-relief treatment and encouraging them to keep themselves as comfortable as possible has several benefits: not surprisingly patients suffer much less postoperative pain. Much less expectedly, on average they actually use a lower total amount of drug than is given when conventional methods are used; perhaps partly as a result of this, they tend to feel ready to go home sooner.

THE PCA SYSTEM

The syringe pump attached to your drip puts you in charge of the process. Your anaesthetist has programmed its computer so that when you press the button twice in quick succession a small amount of pain-relieving drug will be given through the drip. It will work more quickly than the usual sort of injection that is given into a muscle. Nevertheless, its full effects are not apparent for several minutes, and therefore the computer will not give you another dose until a safe time has passed, even if you press the switch again. This means you cannot overdose yourself. It may take several doses to get you comfortable at the beginning; after this you will quickly get used to realizing when the effects are beginning to wear off. It is better to give yourself another dose as soon as this happens; DO NOT wait until you are in a lot of pain. It is also a very good idea to give yourself a dose a few minutes before some event that is likely to prove painful, such as getting out of bed, having physiotherapy, or having a drain removed from the wound. Individuals vary a great deal, and sometimes the dose we choose may make you feel too woozy for a few minutes; if so, tell your nurse and she will get us to try adjusting the dose. Similarly, if the dose we have chosen is too small, you will find that you have to use the button more often than is convenient—again, tell your nurse.

NAUSEA AND SICKNESS

Pain-relieving drugs sometimes make people feel a bit sick, though there is less chance of this with the PCA system. If you do feel at all sick, tell your nurse as soon as possible, as it is best treated early, and a prescription will have been written 'just in case'.

NOISES FROM THE MACHINE

The machine gives a little 'bleep' when you use the button correctly to let you know it has 'got the message': if you don't hear it you may not have pressed hard enough or quickly enough (most of our pumps need you to press twice within one second), so try again, as it won't give you two doses close together. It also has other 'alarm' noises to alert the nurses if, for example, the drip is blocked or the syringe is nearly empty. Do not be worried by these noises: just make sure that they have been noticed by a nurse. The machine is designed to 'fail safe'—if anything at all is wrong it is likely to give you too little drug rather than too much. Therefore it is important to deal with it so that you get good pain relief, but there is no danger if it cannot be sorted out immediately.

FEEDBACK

We would like your comments—ask your nurse for a feedback form or write to me:

Margaret Heath,
Consultant Anaesthetist,
Lewisham Hospital.

6 Understanding PCA equipment

INTRODUCTION

The first commercially available system for allowing patients to use PCA was the Cardiff Palliator (Evans *et al*. 1976). Although no longer manufactured, it is still in use, and was the starting-point from which current machines have been developed. The Cardiff team took a conventional syringe driver and added controls that allow the patient to initiate an injection, the size of which has been pre-set by the anaesthetist. Further controls impose a variable lockout period. Since this depends on a memory facility that is cleared if the power supply is interrupted, it is possible for the lockout period to be circumvented. For this and other reasons substantial design-development has taken place, new manufacturers have entered the market, and choosing the most suitable equipment has become no easy task, particularly in the absence of an independent evaluation programme. We have chosen to concentrate on the equipment normally used for providing PCA in the immediate postoperative period, when the patient is usually in bed. Some of the devices are versatile, and others have been specifically developed for ambulant patients, with a view to their use in chronic pain.

INDEPENDENT EVALUATION

It is a matter of regret that the UK infusion-pump evaluation programme, set up in the early 1980s under the auspices of the Advisory Panel on Anaesthetic Equipment to the then Scientific and Technical Branch of the Department of Health and Social Security, has not been extended to include PCA pumps. An evaluation programme allows dangerous faults to be detected before they pose a hazard, and helpful interaction with manufacturers can lead to responsive development. General guidance on equipment selection and management is available, and those responsible for choosing equipment should study carefully the recommendations of the Medical Devices Directorate of the Department of Health, which are contained in the latest version of *Health Equipment Information* No. 98 (currently November 1990). An evaluation programme could also assist in simplifying some of the procedures required by individual Supplies Departments: the general questionnaire (MLQ declaration) could be greatly reduced in length if the equipment was centrally approved, thus reducing the administrative workload on hospitals and manufacturers. Nevertheless, if the current advice is followed, there should be no question of putting into service a piece of equipment that is electrically or otherwise unsafe, not understood by staff, or unsatisfactory to operate or maintain. Acceptance procedures are of particular importance.

The Emergency Care Research Institute, an independent centre in the USA, has undertaken useful evaluations of a number of PCA pumps (ECRI 1988); these evaluations are only available to subscriber/members however, although some information based on the work has been published recently (Fischberg *et al.* 1991). Since this work was undertaken (before May 1988) considerable changes in design have been made by manufacturers, and the models currently available may have very different performance profiles; the report is nevertheless useful in describing many of the relevant factors that need to be considered.

PUMP-DESIGN DEVELOPMENT

Electronic technological advances have allowed more sophisticated designs to be developed; however, the potential for increased safety has only become a reality somewhat gradually, as malfunction possibilities have also been introduced. Electronic programming may be susceptible to power surges in the electricity supply caused by such events as adjacent lift operation or even plug-removal without switching off. Naturally, designers are alert to these possibilities, and obvious errors are eliminated during design-development. Dangerous possibilities tend only to come to light when very rare combinations of circumstances occur, such as a power surge happening at a precise point in the programming sequence when the machine is set up in a particular and unusual mode. Static electricity has similarly caused extremely rare problems which modification and redesign aim to eliminate.

SUPPLEMENTARY EQUIPMENT

Electronic equipment has to be supplemented by sterile, disposable items to form the drug reservoir and the connection to the patient's intravenous cannula. It was realized early on that simple piggy-backing of PCA on to an existing IV infusion introduced hazards. Avoiding these hazards depends on the availability of a range of suitable items and a thorough understanding of the practicalities of their use.

LEARNING FROM ACCIDENTS

It is to be expected that more widespread usage of PCA will reveal hitherto unexpected dangers, and the existence of a responsive surveillance system to which any such event can be reported is vital. The Medical Devices Directorate of the Department of Health (and similar departments for the NHS outside England) require the reporting of all equipment-related accidents and undertake appropriate investigation in consultation with the manufacturers or suppliers of the equipment. A recent retitling and promotion of the 'NATRIC' (National Reporting and Investigation Centre) has been publized by the Association of Anaesthetists of Great Britain and Ireland. The procedure to be followed is given in the Appendix to Chapter 8. Hospitals must have policies that ensure that all relevant personnel (medical, nursing, pharmacy, electronic/engineering, and administrative) are aware of and have access to the necessary information at all times, day and night. They must also arrange for the regular updating of policies and the issuing of reminders: we suggest that annual provision is necessary. The likelihood of Locum and Agency staff being employed must be taken into account. Few staff will ever activate the system, and therefore a body of knowledge and experience is never developed and passed on; this difference from normal clinical practice is similar to the problems that exist with all rare events. In anaesthetics, the recognition of the importance of prompt, correct action in emergency situations such as failed intubation has made the formulation of protocols and their dissemination commonplace. Administrative actions on which the safety of the wider patient population may depend are no less important.

WHAT IS NEEDED FROM A PCA DEVICE

A. Basic requirements

Box 14. Basic requirements

1. Pre-set bolus dose delivery system
2. Lockout period
3. Provision for prolonged treatment
4. Patient-activation system

The basic requirements for a PCA device include the following features:

1. Ability to deliver an accurate, predetermined bolus dose within a short time-period

In practice, the repeatability with which a set dose is delivered is more important than the absolute accuracy, because the variation in individual requirements is very wide, and the spacing of doses is the principal mechanism by which the patient adjusts dosage-rate to need. If the amount delivered varied greatly it would be more difficult to feel in control, because the effects would be unpredictable. We have no evidence that this is other than a theoretical problem; however, evaluation has shown that accuracy and precision (repeatability) are best when the bolus is contained in a relatively large volume (>0.5 ml), and this will also minimize errors caused by drip occlusion. Devices needing very concentrated solutions are inherently more dangerous, and a balance has to be struck between the desire to avoid frequent refilling and limitation of the total amount of drug within the system. Precision needs to be maintained despite a range of pressures in the patient-delivery system such as may be encountered in normal practice (in the absence of occlusion or clinically important obstruction). This range is likely to be between 5 and 15 kPa. The unit should be capable of delivering the largest bolus volume within one minute. Depending on the configuration of timing controls, longer periods either encroach on the lockout period (reducing safety), or extend it (reducing the availability of drug within a given period).

2. Ability to provide a suitable lockout period

Most of the drugs used for PCA reach their peak effect within a short space of time, and the purpose of the lockout period is to ensure that at least most of the effect of a dose has been appreciated before a further dose can be obtained. Particular situations, such as the commencement of therapy, may require relatively frequent doses, and a three minutes minimum has been suggested as suitable. We would point out, however, that a slow infusion-rate or a large deadspace may effectively reduce the lockout period, and in practice it is rarely advisable to employ less than five minutes. In normal use it is difficult to conceive of the need for lockout periods of as great as twenty minutes; such a length of time significantly reduces the patient's ability to achieve good analgesia, and seems to indicate a reluctance on the part of the prescriber to relinquish control.

3. Ability to operate over a relatively prolonged period

Twenty-four hours is a reasonable minimum, and this places a requirement on both the power source and the size of the drug reservoir. Although battery operation appears attractive from the point of view of mobility, the cost, size, and weight of suitable batteries is often a disadvantage. Exclusively battery-powered equipment is dependent on a 'battery low' alarm which has an unattractive predilection for activation in the early hours of the morning that is possibly related to temperature sensitivity. In general, mains operation with automatic battery back-up for use during transport or when being programmed away from the patient has proved most satisfactory. The equipment should indicate clearly when the battery is in use, and should signal the need for recharging well before exhaustion. The elimination of the need for an electrical power source by using the elastomeric recoil of a silastic drug reservoir has also proved satisfactory and reliable.

4. An activator suitable for patient use in the postoperative period

The mechanism needs to be easy for the patient to operate, but difficult to activate accidentally. It should not get lost or out of reach of the patient, and should give an indication of successful operation. It should be clearly identifiable, with no likelihood of confusion with other equipment: we are amazed at the complacency with which switches virtually identical to nurse-call switches are regarded. Over-dosage has already been reported as a result of the patient's mistaking the demand button for the nurse-call button (Farmer and Harper 1992). Sooner or later an unrelated emergency will be compounded by an extra bolus of analgesic delivered when a visitor assumes he or she is summoning help. We favour the requirement for two presses in quick succession for successful activation: not only does this make accidental activation virtually impossible, but patients can be reassured that a single accidental press will not deliver a dose. It would make random frequent pressing by a confused patient less likely to lead to maximal dosing—a situation which severely tests the ability of sedation to function as the ultimate fail-safe feature of PCA (Stack and Massey 1990). It would also eliminate the possibility of activation caused by the pendant falling to the floor: such an event has been reported (Owen *et al.* 1986), and is made more likely by designs where the button sticks out from the casing; a flat or even recessed design is preferable. Special consideration may be needed for children, for patients with particular handicaps, or for patients undergoing certain types of surgery, for instance on the upper limb. Activators that can be comfortably fixed to the patient in some way avoid the otherwise common problem of the button's getting lost or out of the patient's reach—the Tantalus situation.

B. Additional features

Additional features can be classified into those directed towards patient safety, those directed towards drug security, and those directed towards effectiveness and flexibility in usage; there is inevitably a degree of overlap within these classes: for example, a lockable cover which prevents removal of the drug syringe (a security feature) will also protect the patient from accidental alteration of pump settings (a safety feature).

Box 15. Categories of additional features

1. Safety
2. Security
3. Flexibility
4. Convenience and information

---

1. Patient safety features

i. Program design Design features which favour safety include explicit programming prompts in a logical sequence, with bolus setting corresponding to the dose of drug in mass units (milligrams) rather than as a volume. The chief area in which PCA can endanger the patient is in the preparation of the drug syringe and the programming of the pump. The possibility of error in calculating the initial drug concentration is not totally avoidable, and is discussed in Chapter 8; however, the second calculation involved in translating a bolus dose in milligrams into a volume in millilitres can be assigned to the computer facility of the pump, which is intrinsically more reliable for this particular function than the human brain. Mistakes in calculations of this type are habitually of order differences: for example, the drug syringe contains 10 mg/ml, the bolus prescription is for 2 mg, and the required volume is set for 2 ml rather than 0.2 ml, resulting in a tenfold overdosage.

ii. Overinfusion protection Protection from volume overinfusion as a result of equipment failure or damage can be to some extent incorporated in system design either by flow-limitation or by the requirement for dedicated disposables with suitable characteristics. Antisyphon devices are designed to prevent free flow of solution into the patient should the syringe become detached from the drive mechanism or should air be allowed to enter the system through a defect—usually a crack in a glass vial or syringe. They are basically 'chokes' or flow-restrictors that require a minimum force in excess of that likely to be produced by either the height of the column of fluid or the weight of the syringe plunger or a combination of the two. Glass containers, because of their weight and fragility, are much more vulnerable to syphonage problems, and systems using them require this protection. The relative advantages and disadvantages of plastic and glass containers are discussed later in this chapter. Positive engagement of the plunger by the drive mechanism, with alarm warning of failure, is valuable as an antisyphon safety feature. The use of elastomeric recoil against a choke as the driving power makes syphoning impossible.

iii. Time-period drug limit Early on in treatment, when the patient may have a very low blood level of drug, frequent bolus availablity is desirable to allow rapid control of pain. This has led to the suggestion that the lockout interval appropriate to this situation might allow excessive dosage in the later stages of therapy, and additional controls have been added to some pumps to limit overall consumption within a given time-period (one or four hours). We believe that this conflicts with the basic principle on which the success of PCA is founded—that of patient judgement of dose requirements—and that these alarms are not logical additions to the system; indeed, if they lead to the prescription of inadequate lockout times they could, in susceptible patients, adversely affect safety by allowing repeat doses before the full effects of the initial dose have become apparent. In addition, the very wide variation in sensitivity to opiates means that using an average value for a safe amount will still leave some patients vulnerable to overdosage. The time-period dose limit is most likely to preclude good analgesia when set to levels that accord with the traditional view of opiate dosage: inability of professionals to believe that patients can judge their own needs is, after all, the major problem that remains to be overcome. Worse, an otherwise sensible programme can be wrecked by a simple error in this setting. Farmer and Harper (1992) report three instances of disastrously inadequate analgesia resulting from a four-hour limit setting of 1 mg (presumably as part of a standard 1 mg morphine bolus regime).

iv. Program access Programming systems must be user-friendly; but that very attribute may tempt staff who do not adequately understand either the apparatus or the therapeutic requirements to make alterations rather than to call the appropriate person. Programmable devices should therefore only be accessible to authorized personnel, and a key or password mechanism is necessary to protect the patient from unauthorized changes to the settings. Two-tier programming, with institutional choices for certain basic parameters being incorporated at a higher security level, is a worthwhile sophistication, since it can also reduce the complexity of routine program setting.

v. Instructions for use The clearer the instructions for setting up the apparatus, particularly where electronic programming is needed, the less likelihood of error. We would also make a plea for simplicity. An individual user's whim may become incorporated into pump design in the hope that it will prove to be a selling-point. Complexity is offputting to the ordinary user, however, and may reduce safety by increasing the possibility of misunderstanding. Most institutions wisely aim to standardize their regimens to some degree, and the introduction of two-tier programming may resolve this dilemma.

2. Security features

PCA systems inevitably contain substantial amounts of narcotic drugs. There is no way round this basic fact if they are to serve the purpose of making pain relief available for at least twenty-four hours to patients, some of whom will have high requirements. There is therefore a potential security problem, which can only partly be addressed by machine design. Other aspects of security are considered in the sections on supervision (Chapter 11), protocols, and documentation (Chapter 9). Design solutions can include locking devices which secure the drug reservoir within the machine and/or the machine to the infusion stand. Alarms can be provided which can only be disabled by key or password. The security requirement is then passed on to the key- or password-holder, and this is likely to diminish its effectiveness, as convenience demands easy availability: the key may be attached to the pump, or the password may become known to all ward staff.

3. Features promoting effectiveness and flexibility in use

i. Occlusion alarms To be effective, a PCA system clearly must generate sufficient power to overcome the maximum normally encountered resistance of the intravenous cannula combined with intravascular pressure (unlikely to exceed 25 kPa). Beyond this basic requirement it is possible to seek to enhance effectiveness by warning if excessive resistance, denoting occlusion of the cannula (or other other line obstruction), is present. This should ensure that therapy is not interrupted, thus avoiding a fall in blood drug concentration and loss of confidence in the system. Although major backing-up of drug into the infusion line is precluded by use of a one-way (anti-reflux) valve or a dedicated cannula, occlusion of the cannula can still lead to the storing-up of small volumes under pressure. The size of this effect is determined by the distensibility of the system, and the degree of hazard depends on the concentration of drug in the solution. The lack of drug effect will lead to repeated demands, and the equivalent of several doses may be delivered if the occlusion is released without disconnecting the patient; this alarm therefore also has safety implications. The choice of the pressure at which such an alarm is activated is a balance between minimizing this possibility and avoiding over-frequent alarm signals when the cannula is temporarily occluded by patient movement. A maximum pressure for occlusion alarm triggering of 100 kPa has recently been recommended (Fischberg *et al.* 1991). Non-distensible delivery systems, power-limitation of the delivery system (so that drug cannot be pushed out against resistances that are significantly higher than normal), and relatively large bolus volumes (implying low drug concentrations) reduce the need for occlusion alarms from a safety point of view.

ii. Reservoir-refilling alert This is a helpful feature for similar reasons to those for occlusion alarms: if the device signals the need to recharge the syringe (preferably before it is totally empty) therapy will not be interrupted. Proper supervision and monitoring of patients and their rates of drug demand (which tend to be relatively stable) should ensure that the drug supply is replenished at suitable convenient times without an alarm, although there may be occasions when the rate of drug consumption alters abruptly; this should be a signal to look for some adverse event, such as the development of surgical complications.

iii. Background infusion facility A facility for background infusions which allows continuous delivery of drug theoretically provides for less fluctuation of blood levels and therefore of pain relief. In practice (as we discussed in Chapter 3), the use of such infusions has not fulfilled expectations, although they are likely to prove useful in special circumstances. Developments such as patient-controlled epidural analgesia seem a probable area of application.

iv. Variable bolus volume Standardization of drug concentration is a worthwhile way of reducing errors in fulfilling prescriptions, and, as many adult patients can be managed very satisfactorily with a standard bolus dose, it is possible to provide a good service with a single bolus volume. Nevertheless, the extreme variability of drug requirement means that the ability to vary the bolus dose by varying the volume delivered is a great advantage, since a significant proportion of patients (especially if children are included in the service) may otherwise require a non-standard drug concentration. It has been suggested that a range from 0.5 ml to 5.0 ml is required (Fischberg *et al*. 1991). There is something to be said for a somewhat smaller range, since this could alert the person programming the pump to a potentially dangerous tenfold error: failure to complete the program for a bolus that would require 5 ml of solution when 0.5 ml was intended should lead to reassessment of the calculation. Bolus volumes below 0.5 ml are susceptible to lack of accuracy and precision; they also lead to the use of concentrated solutions, which are more dangerous if accidental overinfusion occurs; and it is our view that they should not be used routinely, and perhaps should not be available.

v. Variable dose-delivery rate   Some pumps allow slower than standard delivery rates to be chosen. These might conceivably be useful where a large volume is being delivered into a small vein; in practice they are rarely if ever used. Bolus doses that are large enough to cause unwanted systemic effects are unlikely to be made much more acceptable by reducing the rate of delivery, unless it is slowed to the point where the length of time will have to be taken into account when setting the lockout period.

vi. Displays of program, demands, and dosage   The point of PCA is to allow patients to determine how much drug they receive, and it might therefore be argued that simple labelling of the drug reservoir and appropriate documentation of drug consumption on the prescription chart is all that is required. There is no doubt in our minds, however, that the ability to display and review the program of an electronic pump is vital to the safe and effective management of patients. It is also valuable, both for individual patient care and for cumulative experience, to be able to see easily how many demands the patient has made and how much drug has been delivered. Patients' perceptions of the appropriateness of the bolus size and how often they have to push the button are the most important factors in reviewing whether changes in the regimen are needed; nevertheless, most patients are very unwilling to complain or cause any sort of trouble, and the provision of information greatly assists staff in optimizing treatment. It is particularly helpful if the information on drug consumption and the programmed regime are not cleared when the unit is turned off or the power supply is interrupted, since full documentation may not have been completed. Clearing the information from the last patient should be a preliminary part of the programming routine.

vii. Signals for the patient's benefit   It is reassuring to the patient (and the staff) if an audible signal is generated when a demand is made. If the machine also indicates whether it is able to respond to a demand, i.e. whether it is within the lockout period, patients who seek the maximum control by interacting intelligently with the system can decide, for instance, to give themselves two doses within a minimum period prior to potentially painful events such as getting out of bed or having physiotherapy. It should be remembered, however, that patients receiving opiates who have also had a general anaesthetic quite recently will not be totally clear-headed. The green light indicating the availability of a bolus has been misunderstood as a positive instruction to activate the machine (Johnson and Daugherty 1992), with resultant oversedation.

viii. Alarm disablement   Audible alarms should be appropriately pitched, so that they are noticed but do not engender panic. It should not be possible permanently to silence an alarm intended to protect the patient from a serious hazard without either correcting the fault or ensuring the patient's safety in some other way. That said, there is no doubt that the quality of the alarm system in terms of appropriateness, controllability, and comprehensibility is a key feature in staff acceptance of apparatus.

ix. Hard-copy record   Information held within an electronic pump's memory can be downloaded by interfacing with a suitable printer. The format of printouts rarely makes them easy to file in the patient's notes or particularly useful clinically. Whilst it is possible that such records might have medicolegal value, properly kept manual records are in any case essential. Printouts may be judged valuable for research purposes, particularly since they may reduce the effects of observer error or bias.

x. Disposable recognition/dedication   Equipment requiring additional disposables such as syringes and lines may be designed for use only with specific items, alternatives giving rise to problems with accuracy or security. Such equipment should 'recognize' incorrect items either by physical blocks to fitting or by registering an alarm message. Clearly, the ability to use any make of suitably-sized syringe is an advantage. Sophisticated equipment that can be programmed to accept whichever disposable syringe is institutionally available can minimize running costs without restricting flexibility should contracts change.

xi. General convenience   Finally, the weight and size of a machine and the flexibility with which it can be positioned can greatly affect the convenience of staff and therefore its overall acceptability on a crowded, busy surgical ward. Robustness of construction and security of attachment of leads and controls are similarly very important practical considerations. Owen *et al.* (1986) describe an 'unplanned' test in which a machine survived a fall of 0.9 m. Life is full of such tests, and terrazzo flooring is unforgiving.

SUPPLEMENTARY EQUIPMENT

It is possible for a sterile disposable unit to be connected directly to a dedicated cannula and thus provide PCA without any additional specialized items. In all other circumstances additional equipment is needed which must satisfy standard requirements for sterility, connections, packaging, etc.

i. One-way valves

If a unit is to be connected to the side port of a coexisting intravenous infusion, an anti-reflux valve is required to prevent the retrograde passage of a delivered dose into the infusion set in the event of occlusion of the outflow to the patient. Without it, repeated demands lead to the accumulation of large amounts of analgesic that will enter the patient's circulation rapidly if the obstruction is cleared without disconnection. This danger is explained in more detail in Chapter 8 (see Figs. 8.1–8.4, pp. 107–11). Valves need to have a low compliance (be non-distensible) so that they are not themselves capable of storing significant quantities of fluid when pressurized. They need to have low internal volumes, since they act as additional deadspace in the system which, with slow infusion rates, will delay the delivery of drug to the patient; this can have two undesirable effects: delay in obtaining analgesia and encroachment on the lockout period, which could lead to an additional demand's being made before the full effects of the first have developed. The design should minimize the possibility of misconnection, and not reduce unduly the infusion flow-rate.

ii. Drug reservoirs

Standard-pattern disposable plastic syringes are accurate, cheap, and readily available. Many of the syringe drivers that have been modified to produce programmable PCA pumps use them as a routine. Although they are not intended for prolonged contact with drug solutions there is very little evidence of problems resulting from their use with the common analgesic agents. Adsorption is maximal within the first three hours, and can be of the order of 10 per cent (Duthie *et al*. 1987). Thereafter, little change can be detected, and the differences have not proved to be clinically significant. Their strength and lightness together with the relatively high friction between plunger and barrel make their use less likely to lead to syphoning accidents as a result either of cracks that allow air to enter or plunger descent if detachment from the drive mechanism occurs.

Glass vials or syringes allow prolonged storage, and therefore can be commercially prepared, possibly reducing one element of hazard. The lower frictional forces also allow lower settings on occlusion alarms, which may be perceived as an advantage.

The silastic drug reservoir used to generate the infusion force in the only disposable PCA device currently available has proved robust and exhibits similar characteristics with regard to the adsorption of analgesic drugs to those of plastic syringes. Whilst clinically insignificant, the differences in the concentration of drug delivered may need to be borne in mind when studies of systems using glass vials or syringes are compared with those using plastic or silastic drug reservoirs.

We favour large drug reservoirs (50–60 ml) to reduce the number of times recharging is required without forcing the use of concentrated solutions and small bolus volumes.

iii. Connecting lines and anti-syphon devices

We have taken the view that connecting lines need to be stiff-walled, of low internal volume, and non-kinking, so that they contribute minimally to the distensibility of the system, and cannot be obstructed by external forces. However, some manufacturers offer soft-walled lines with clamp devices, so that the line can be deliberately occluded when the syringe is changed to avoid accidental administration of drug solution. This complicates the syringe-changing routine, and, if the clamp is accidentally left on, will lead to activation of the occlusion alarm (if present) or to non-delivery of a bolus when the patient next requests one. Whichever type is chosen, the choice must be adhered to and explicitly taken account of in the syringe-changing instructions. If the non-kinking type is chosen, care must be taken when inserting the new syringe in the driving mechanism so that extra drug is not accidentally infused. If soft-walled lines with clamps are in use, clear instructions may be given to clamp the line at the start and to remember to unclamp it at the finish. Anti-syphon devices need to provide a reliable resistance to flow appropriate to the particular pump design, ensuring that only pump operation will deliver drug to the patient. Recently introduced connecting lines combining anti-syphon and anti-back-up valves are the safest choice, although they increase costs.

WHAT IS AVAILABLE

At the time of writing, manufacturers/distributors are offering the following models:

Abbott: Lifecare PCA Infusion pump;

Bard: PCA I pump (they also market the Ambulatory PCA pump, which we have not used);

Baxter: PCA Infuser system: 5 ml/hr, (there is also a 2 ml/hr version which we have not used); and

Graseby: 3300 Syringe pump.

However, earlier devices (the Cardiff 'Palliator' and the Graseby PCAS) are still in use in many hospitals, and are therefore included in this descriptive section.

Cardiff 'Palliator' (Fig. 6.1)

This first PCA machine has stood the test of time remarkably well. It requires a 30 ml syringe, and is programmed by setting rotating switches at the back of the machine to indicate the rate of infusion, the lockout interval, and the concentration of solution used. The latter is unfortunately required in microlitres per milligram—an unconventional system which is extremely confusing. Bolus dose is set in milligrams on the front panel, and is released in response to a pneumatic handswitch which must be depressed twice within one second, but is otherwise identical to that supplied with the Graseby PCAS (see below). The lockout interval depends on a memory which is wiped by interruption of the mains supply, and it is therefore theoretically possible for it to be circumvented. It will be cleared during transfer of the patient; but the time taken for this is very unlikely to be less than the lockout period, and has never led to a clinical problem. The front panel displays the total dosage adminis tered since reset. The machine does not lock, and is therefore vulnerable to unauthorized reprogramming and to theft of the

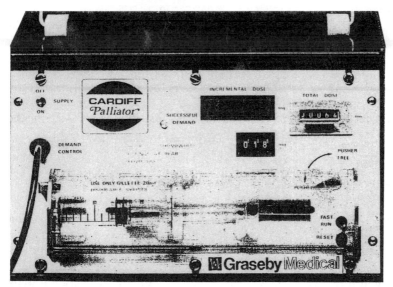

Fig. 6.1. The Cardiff 'Palliator'.

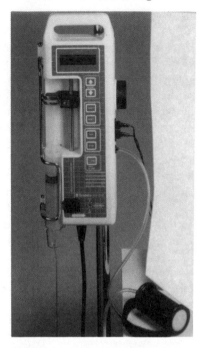

Fig. 6.2. The Graseby PCAS.

drug syringe. Despite this, and its weight and bulk (5.6 kg, 310 mm × 210 mm × 205 mm) it works well on wards with good observation and nurses experienced in looking after patients on PCA.

Graseby PCAS (Fig. 6.2)

The Graseby Patient Controlled Analgesia System is a development of a syringe pump that has been in wide use for some years. It is designed to take a standard 50/60 ml syringe (BD Plastipak), which is locked into the drive system. It is mains-powered, with back-up internal rechargeable batteries, and can be clamped to drip-stand or trolley-rail. Programming requires key release, is menu-driven, and requests either variation or confirmation of drug concentration, bolus dose, loading dose, infusion rate, background infusion, and lockout interval. Bolus doses are released following a single depression of the flush-set button of the pneumatic handset, which has a Velcro strap for the patient's hand. Each press (whether 'successful', i.e. outside the lockout period, or not) is accompanied by a beep. The display records total dosage since programming. The unit weighs 2.75 kg and measures 366 mm × 127 mm × 80 mm. Successive modification of the software has been undertaken to eliminate problems caused by power surges and static accumulation.

Abbott Lifecare PCA Infusion Pump (Fig. 6.3)

This machine takes a standard Becton Dickinson 30 ml luerlock syringe which locks into the drive mechanism (alarm sounds if improperly positioned). Security is excellent. Programming is menu-driven with a large (too large, in our opinion) number of options. The purge facility is clearly a possible source of danger if the instruction to disconnect from the patient is ignored or overlooked.

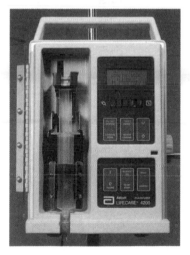

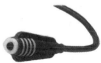

Fig. 6.3. The Abbott PCA Plus.

The patient switch resembles a nurse-call button, projecting from its casing; it releases a bolus in response to a single press. The unit is relatively heavy and bulky (7 kg, 210 mm × 340 mm × 150 mm), and this, combined with the multiplicity of alarms, does not endear it to nursing staff.

Bard PCA 1 Pump (Fig. 6.4)

Rotating dial switches are used to simplify programming of this device, which takes a 60 ml luerlock syringe. This limits the flexibility of dosage and lockout time (designated 'delay') somewhat, and

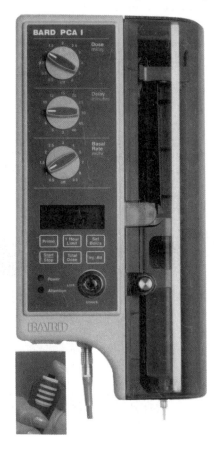

Fig. 6.4. The Bard PCA 1.

means that programming is a mixture of menu- and switch-setting. More serious disadvantages are the use of a volumetric dose and the confusing display panel, which uses a mix of upper- and lower-case letters. The word 'bolus' is used unconventionally for a loading dose, and not for the dose for self-administration. The batteries, used as the sole power source, are both heavy and expensive.

Baxter PCA Infusor (Fig. 6.5)

This disposable device comes as two presterilized units: the Infusor and the Patient Control Module (PCM). The Infusor consists of an elastomeric balloon reservoir which is charged by attaching a luerlock syringe (normally 50/60 ml, but could be 30 ml) filled with opiate at a concentration that contains the required bolus dose in 0.5 ml. Once chosen, this bolus dose can only be altered by replacing the Infusor with another one charged with a different concentration of drug. The force (not inconsiderable) taken to distend the balloon provides the motive power for infusion. A

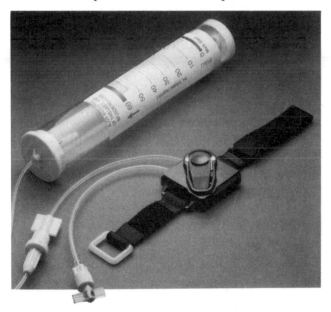

Fig. 6.5. The Baxter PCA Infusor.

choke built into the delivery line restricts output to a constant 5 ml per hour, and this is used to prime the line and the PCM—this operation cannot therefore be hurried; the constant infusion rate determines the lockout period, since it takes 6 minutes to fill or refill the bolus dose reservoir in the PCM. The PCM has a springloaded switch that releases its 0.5 ml reservoir via a short connecting line to the IV cannula; it resembles a wristwatch with a Velcro strap, and is normally worn by the patient on the side on which the cannula is sited, and operated by depressing the switch with the other hand. If the site of surgery precludes this arrangement we find it easiest to position the strap round the fingers, so that the patient can depress the switch with the thumb of the same hand. The Infusor is extremely light, and can be pinned to the patients' clothing. It is difficult to see that a dose has been delivered, and there is, of course, no record of failed attempts; neither is it easy (because of parallax between the paper strip and the volume indicator) to be sure of the total dose delivered. Nevertheless the system works very well in practice, and is particularly liked by patients: it obviously has a much less 'high-tech' appearance than the electronic pumps.

Graseby 3300 (Fig. 6.6)

This relatively new addition to the range combines sophistication with simplicity by providing two-tier programming. An exceptionally full range of options for background infusion, loading dose, speed of infusion, etc, etc. is available by 'unlocking' the program using a combination of keys. Once options have been selected and 'locked', daily operation can be reduced to a simple menu-driven program confined to drug concentration, bolus dose, and lockout time. The machine will accept commonly available disposable 30 or 60 ml syringes, and senses the type as well as the correct location within the drive mechanism. It employs the traditional pneumatic handset, which some patients find difficult to operate, especially in the early stages. Recently, a new handset has been designed which is a great deal easier to use, and retains the important feature of a flush switch. The Velcro strap has been replaced by a wrist loop that appears to work well as a retainer. The unit can be clamped to drip-stand or trolley, but will also sit on any convenient horizontal surface. The accompanying documentation is clear and well presented. The unit weighs 3 kg and measures 334 mm × 195 mm × 130 mm, and is mains-driven with battery back-up.

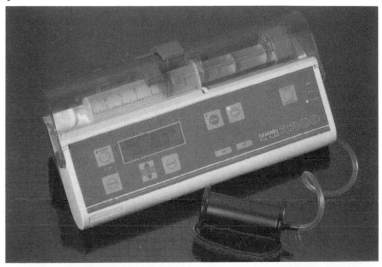

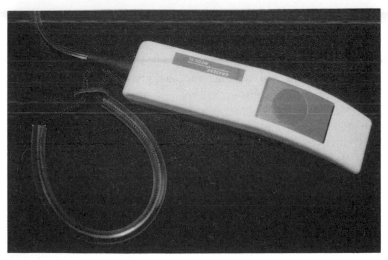

Fig. 6.6. The Graseby 3300 PCA Pump, with its new handset, which can also be fitted to the Graseby PCAS.

Box 16. Features of currently available PCA systems

Make/model	Palliator	Graseby PCAS	Bard	Baxter	Graseby 3300	Abbott
power source (mains/battery)	M	M/B	B	NA	M/B	M/B
weight	u	++	+	+++	++	u
general convenience of fixing, etc.	u	++	++	+++	++	+
security	u	++	+++	+	+++	+++
ease of programming	+	++	+	NA	+++	++
flexibility of bolus	+	+++	++	NA	+++	+++
flexibility of lockout	+	+++	++	NA	+++	+++
activation switch	++	++	u	+++	++	u
alarm messages	NA	+++	+	NA	+++	+++
user instructions	NA	+++	++	+++	+++	+++
additional features		abcd fgh	bcd fgh		abcd efgh	abcd efgh
undesirable features		y	xyz		xy	xyz

KEY: u = unsatisfactory, + = satisfactory, ++ = good, +++ = very good. NA = not applicable/available

additional features: a   printer available
                       b   background infusion option
                       c   history review

                       alarms: d   occlusion
                                 e   syringe placement
                                 f   low/empty syringe
                                 g   low battery
                                 h   system/mains failure

undesirable features: x   purge option
                        y   loading dose
                        z   dedicated disposables recommended

We have not carried out systematic laboratory evaluations of PCA equipment. All pumps that we have used on patients have satisfied the electrical safety requirements and tests of accuracy applied by our hospital electronics department. One make of pump, the Bionica MDS 110 (not currently available) gave rise to a substantial overdose (and a Hazard Notice) when the drive disconnected from the syringe plunger and the weight of the glass plunger both provided its own driving force and allowed syphonage (Grover and Heath 1992).

7 What makes PCA safe?

We have outlined the reasons for regarding PCA as a significant advance in managing postoperative pain when compared with the methods in more general use: regular or on-demand intramuscular opiates, continuous IV infusions, and oral analgesics.

Box 17. Safety factors with PCA

- Patient activation—conscious decision and effort required
- Intravenous route—rapid onset of effects
- Small individual dose—no depot effect
- Lower average total dose—but greater efficacy
- Reduced number of prescription events

Before any care team introduces a new method of caring for its patients, a major consideration has to be safety. However, nurses and doctors are resistant to change: it disturbs their comfortable routines, and concern with safety may sometimes appear to be a strategy directed against innovation. Let us reject that unworthy premiss and examine first of all the theoretical basis for recommending PCA as an acceptably safe method of postoperative pain management in the real world in which we work—NHS hospitals in the United Kingdom of the 1990s. The basic principle of PCA, that of the patient's initiating the administration of the drug, is the first safety feature. The human animal is intelligent, and most patients are extremely unlikely to give themselves a dose of something that they know is potent and possibly dangerous unless they have good reasons. More important than that, however, is the fact that if they fall asleep or are oversedated (not always easily distinguishable states) they simply will not activate the machine, and are thus protected.

The intravenous route ensures reliable and rapid onset of effect. When an intramuscular injection is given, absorption into the blood must precede any clinical effect, and therefore variability in absorption as well as the finite time that it takes are important factors. The principal components of variability are the site of the injection (both the actual muscle and the depth within it have been shown to affect the rate of absorption of drugs) and the state of the circulation. Even in one patient, the depth and site of injection and the circulatory state on which absorption is also dependent may vary markedly from one administration to another. The particular-time period during which careful observation may be important cannot be predicted with any accuracy, and, the drug effect being both delayed and more prolonged compared with that via the intravenous route, the observer is more vulnerable to distraction. Peak blood levels in uncomplicated postoperative patients in one study were found to be reached anywhere between 20 and 100 minutes (Austin *et al.* 1980*b*). It is obvious that a patient with poor peripheral circulation may absorb drug more slowly than usual; but it is fairly surprising that injecting morphine intramuscularly into gluteus maximus whilst the patient is under spinal blockade appears also to delay absorption, the mean peak effect occuring at 90 min, with substantial inter-patient variability in blood levels (Kay *et al.* 1985). Eliminating this variability contributes greatly to safety: during the initial period of stabilization of a patient on PCA there is no doubt in the minds of supervisory staff about the need to observe patients carefully immediately after a dose has been taken—but for a relatively short length of time. With an intramuscular injection, a nurse may feel (with reasonable confidence) that not a lot will happen for at least 15 minutes; it is clearly somewhat optimistic to expect her to remember to start observing the patient then and for perhaps up to two hours to detect peak effects. It is important to realize that the absence of a depot of the drug gives PCA two further safety features: any adverse event caused by idiosyncracy will be relatively evanescent, and serious change in patient sensitivity resulting from general deterioration (for example as a result of haemorrhage) will tend to be limited. By contrast, relentless continued absorption from an intramuscular injection site will require greater corrective action in these circumstances. Our experience has been mainly with papaveretum, a drug mixture of which the active analgesic component is morphine, probably the slowest-acting of the drugs used for PCA (because of its lower lipid-solubility). A study of respiratory effects (Annan *et al.* 1988) has shown that, whilst the greater part of the effect on depth of breathing following IV morphine is evident after 1.5 minutes, respiratory rate takes a little longer (around 3 minutes); the same study showed that diamorphine, expected on theoretical grounds to be quicker in onset, probably does not differ significantly from morphine.

Doubling these times for safety still produces a timescale which makes observation during the clinically important period a realistic probability. Moreover, nurses can feel confident about when to stop watching closely in a way that cannot be assured after intramuscular injections. In addition, the intravenous route eliminates many of the variables that can affect the response to individual doses: this lessens the likelihood of any dangerous change in sensitivity. The study referred to above was performed in lightly anaesthetized, unstimulated patients; however, many of the studies laying stress on the respiratory-depressant potential of the opiate drugs have been performed on volunteers without pain, and their relevance to the clinical situation is far from clear. Experience suggests that clinically significant respiratory depression will normally be obvious within five minutes and, conversely, that depression not obvious at that time rarely worsens to the point of significance.

Most clinical experience with PCA in the UK has been with papaveretum, diamorphine, or morphine (Cartwright *et al.* 1991; Notcutt and Morgan 1990; Wheatley *et al.* 1991), and confirms the basic safety of the technique. Other drugs that have been widely used for PCA are fentanyl and pethidine. Both these have an even more rapid onset of effects (including of course respiratory depression), and this profile is one of the features that is advantageous from a safety aspect. The increasing use of pulse oximetry within recovery rooms will allow a much better appreciation of mild respiratory depression and validation (or otherwise) of these statements in the context of routine clinical practice. In addition, simple respiratory monitors are being developed which will be able to supplement intermittent observation. The fact that patients tend to establish their own rate of drug usage relatively early (Hull and Sibbald 1981) may allow us to identify the very occasional patient (for example those with unappreciated respiratory disease) in whom mild respiratory depression causes unacceptable hypoxia despite an apparently satisfactory PCA regime (Wheatley *et al.* 1992). These patients will require more complex methods of pain relief, and a higher intensity of observation, monitoring, and treatment: identifying them during the early recovery period will make it easier to optimize their care. This study highlighted the fact that patients undergoing abdominal surgery are more at risk from conventional intramuscular on-demand opiate therapy. Another study from the same group (Madej *et al*. 1992) confirmed this, and showed similar dangers from epidural opiate analgesia: it did not prove possible to predict those most at risk by preoperative observation.

The PCA regime, by allowing patients to adjust their own drug requirements, results in a lower total drug consumption than standard on-demand IM injections for a given level of pain relief. This has been shown by a study in our hospital which compared patients having similar operations, nursed on the same ward and comparable for age, weight, and psychological profile (Thomas *et al*. 1990). Some early studies found that PCA increased the amount of drug administered to the patients. These results almost certainly reflect the common problems associated with nurse-administered IM opiates: the effects of cautious prescribing and the timing delays and communication difficulties which in reality reduce the amount of drug available to the patient. Once ward staff have seen the results obtainable with PCA they become more committed to good pain relief for their patients, however prescribed: this led to many patients on the standard regime in our study being given the maximum dosage allowed by the prescriber. Relatively poor results in the IM group despite this emphasize the inability of the anaesthetist accurately to predict individual dose requirements.

Reduced total dosage has obvious advantages for safety, both in normal circumstances and in situations where abnormal sensitivities, circulatory failure, metabolic pathway overload, or drug interactions may arise during treatment.

Within any hospital system caring for large numbers of acute patients, prescription and administration errors do occur, albeit infrequently, despite well-established protocols for calculating, drawing up, and checking both drug and patient. The institution of PCA reduces the liability to such errors by reducing the number of procedures and situations where such errors can occur: the vast majority of patients will be satisfactorily managed on the initial prescription because the variation in dose requirement is regulated by the patient. In addition, many patients will not require more than one charging of the drug reservoir, and therefore the number of times a potentially dangerous interpretation of a prescription and connection to the drug-delivery system occurs is very greatly reduced; in particular the number of such activities carried out at night and by staff not familiar with the patient or the immediate perioperative condition is reduced. The close observation possible in recovery and high-dependency areas, where the immediate effects of any such mistakes should become apparent and where PCA is routinely commenced, add a further degree of patient safety.

Technological advances have allowed the design of PCA systems to evolve, improving reliability and eliminating sources of machine malfunction, some of which have arisen because of unusual combinations of circumstances. The Medical Devices Directorate of the Department of Health has overall responsibility for monitoring the safety of patient-related equipment in England and Wales (similar arrangements, with interdepartmental communication, exist for Scotland and Northern Ireland). Any event demonstrating a possible hazard must be reported with appropriate urgency; investigation is undertaken in consultation with the manufacturers of the device, and action is instituted according to the results. Issue of a Hazard Notice and withdrawal of apparatus may be undertaken pending design modification, or a Safety Information Bulletin may be published giving advice to users on how to avoid hazardous situations. It is often found that user error, arising from either ignorance or misunderstanding, or deliberate contravention of the instructions for proper use, is the root cause of accidents. The procedure for notification of such incidents is detailed in the appendix to Chapter 8. The number of incidents related to PCA referred to the Department of Health for investigation during recent years is reassuringly low at approximately three per year, and few incidents have been reported within the international literature in recent years, despite increasing use of the system. Clearly the level of observation is crucial to safety, and the wider introduction of high-dependency units with a level of staffing similar to that of recovery units, but where patients can stay for 24–48 hours after major surgery has been advocated (Association of Anaesthetists of Great Britain and Ireland 1991). On present experience PCA appears to be safe on postoperative wards where patients can have good general observation and regular checks of physiological parameters as dictated by their surgical condition. No patient should be placed in a single room nor equivalent visual isolation if they are to have a reasonable chance of surviving **any** sudden catastrophe, whether it be pulmonary embolism or PCA pump malfunction, and sudden dangerous changes in post-surgical condition must be acknowledged to be more likely within the first 2–3 days; the cost-effectiveness of higher levels of observation will be difficult to sustain, given the very low incidence of accidents and the high level of safety of the method in normal use.

Both we and the manufacturers of pump systems would emphasize that staff training and familiarization are essential, and that meticulous attention to information and understanding, and to protocols for prescription and the preparation and connection of systems must be maintained.

8 Sources of danger to the patient

INTRODUCTION

It is as well to attempt to enumerate all the possible sources of danger to the patient that are inherent in the use of PCA. Many of them are common to other forms of postoperative analgesia, but a thorough appraisal may help users to recognize and adopt the appropriate safeguards within their own actions and to encourage and support their colleagues in maintaining safe practice. Inevitably, much of the content of this chapter can also be found in the individual sections on drugs, equipment, and patient-related aspects of PCA; however, given the way that human error seems to permeate through most of the problems, we have here adopted a chronological approach, which highlights the frequency with which interacting factors operate.

Box 18. Sources of danger to the patient

1. Patient selection/education
2. Drug-prescription errors
3. Inappropriate prescribing
4. Programming errors
5. Filling/installing drug reservoir
6. Patient connection
7. Abnormal drug reactions
8. Equipment malfunction
9. Moving patient and/or equipment
10. Non-patient activation
11. Long-term use

---

1. PATIENT SELECTION AND EDUCATION

PCA has been used for an extremely wide range of patients; nevertheless, it is possible to identify preoperatively some classes of patient who are unlikely to use it satisfactorily either for psychological reasons (discussed in Chapter 4) or because of limited intellectual capacity. The anaesthetist, at the preoperative visit, must make a realistic appraisal of the likelihood of a patient's coping with the system. As an example, patients with Alzheimer's disease or other dementias might be expected to be easily recognizable, but, in the early stages, they can maintain an appearance of social functioning based on more-or-less reflex conversational responses that obscures their inability to take in new information. Normally the system will 'fail-safe', since it will not be activated; but there remains a possibility that repeated button pressing might occur, leading to somnolence. This would only become a danger if the bolus dose were on the high side and the lockout interval too short.

Similarly, the capability of children and adolescents must be carefully assessed. No preoperative assessment system will be perfect, and careful supervision in the early postoperative period remains an essential safeguard, since the effects of anaesthetic and sedative drugs on intellectual functioning are not entirely predictable. A case has been described of an adolescent's achieving relative overdosage by repeated button-pressing of which she had no recollection after the event (Stack and Massey 1990). In another incident (Farmer and Harper 1992), a patient mistook the button for the nurse-call button, and repeatedly pressed it until she became comatose. No intervention was deemed necessary, and no permanent harm ensued; but it was clearly an undesirable event, to which unsatisfactory design of the demand button contributed.

Information supplied to patients preoperatively needs to be carefully scrutinized for accuracy and comprehensibility. It seems possible that patients in the future will arrive in hospital with inaccurate knowledge derived from a variety of personal and media sources, as frequently happens in obstetric pain-relief services. Over-elaboration of the possibilities can confuse (Johnson and Daugherty 1992), and it is best to be sure that the basic operation of the system is satisfactory before moving on to more sophisticated routines. Listening to the patient and being alert to such possibilities should isolate any dangers.

2. DRUG PRESCRIPTION ERRORS

Prescription errors will endanger the patient if they lead to single, very large bolus doses. This can happen in two ways: the wrong dose is chosen (perhaps that appropriate for pethidine is used for morphine), or the wrong dilution volume is specified, leading to a higher concentration than intended. The chances of these errors' occurring are minimized by restricting prescribing to practitioners who are familiar with the drugs used and have undergone supervised training within the institution, thus ensuring familiarity with the format of the prescription chart and the volume of the equipment's drug reservoir. Anaesthetists are well placed to fulfil these require-ments, and errors are less likely to be translated into disasters if the prescriber also undertakes the charging of the device. It is however essential that a second person, who is qualified to take charge of controlled drugs and understands the principles of PCA, checks each stage in the preparation of the equipment for use. Standardization of regimes, both in terms of the drug and the dilution used, reduces the likelihood of error. There are advantages in having a purpose-designed prescription chart which leads the prescriber through each step:

'____(total in mass units) of _____(drug) to _____(total volume of drug reservoir) with _____(diluent),
[to produce concentration ____(mass /ml)]
Bolus dose: _____(mass units) [contained in _____ml]'

An example of this type of chart is given in the appendix to Chapter 9.

As PCA becomes a more common mode of postoperative pain relief, it is likely that provision of standardized stock syringes prepared aseptically within the hospital pharmacy or by commercial suppliers will be used to reduce the workload on anaesthetic staff. With proper safeguards, such systems should prove as safe as or safer than individual preparation, and may allow simplification of prescribing regimes.

Errors, as opposed to misjudgements, seem relatively unlikely with respect to prescription of the lockout period. They could occur when setting limits on the drug total available to the patient in a given time-period (a facility on some pumps); however, as was discussed in Chapter 6, the value of this control is marginal, and the combination of bolus dose and lockout period remains the ultimate control on the total quantity of drug available within the prescription. Normally, the patient will not need the total amount, which is thus irrelevant to safety, although, for the occasional very high user, it can be extremely relevant to efficacy and satisfaction.

3. INAPPROPRIATE PRESCRIBING

Choices of drug, and of bolus dose and/or lockout periods that are inappropriate to a particular patient are all possible dangers. The effects of many of the drugs used during anaesthesia last into the recovery period, and may theoretically interact with drugs used for PCA. Respiratory depression has been described relatively late when papaveretum (in a substantial intramuscular dose) is given to patients in whom fentanyl has been used intraoperatively (Adams and Pybus 1978). This is inherently less likely to be a problem with PCA because of the relatively small changes in opiate drug levels that result from its incremental nature. It is also possible that a patient's circulatory state may be so depressed that commonly-used lockout periods prove too short to allow the full effect of a bolus to be revealed. Under normal conditions, the institution of PCA within the well-supervised surroundings of the Recovery area ensures that inappropriate regimes and unstable circulatory or respiratory states are detected and dealt with. Clearly, sudden deterioration of a patient because of the onset of surgical complications later in the postoperative course must pose a hazard; however, once again the small size of individual bolus doses in comparison to those involved in intramuscular regimes makes PCA less hazardous in these circumstances, and problems of this nature have not been serious. Nevertheless, the need for good general observation cannot be overemphasized.

4. INITIAL PROGRAMMING ERRORS

The possibility of gross errors of programming must always lurk in wait for the careless. As with prescribing, restriction to properly trained personnel along with standardized regimes and rigorous checking are the best protection. Logical programming prompts on computerized equipment are easy to achieve, and their desirability should be borne in mind when selecting equipment. It is extremely unlikely that an error in this area will escape detection in the Recovery room, unless the effects of techniques involving local anaesthetics have not been given enough time to wear off.

5. FILLING AND INSTALLING THE DRUG RESERVOIR

This requires following the prescription and, as was discussed above, errors can be introduced if insufficient detail is specified or a second competent person is not available to check each stage. Poor handwriting allows the possibility of misinterpretation. Clearly, bulk preparation of stock syringes has the potential to reduce dilution errors.

Equipment based on a syringe driver requires the syringe to be correctly fitted into and held by the drive mechanism. Failure will usually be indicated by inability to close the cover or to initiate therapy, and some pumps have specific sensors that prevent this error. In one incident, a failure of this type, compounded by the characteristics of the glass syringe, led to the rapid infusion of approximately 180 mg of papaveretum into a patient (Grover and Heath 1992). The patient fortunately suffered no permanent ill effects, and the subsequent investigation resulted in the total withdrawal of the particular model of pump. More thorough independent evaluation of PCA devices before they are marketed, and especially after any modifications are introduced, is essential to reduce equipment-related hazards. Syphonage from a cracked glass reservoir allowing air to enter is more likely if the reservoir is placed very high. It is good practice always to place the reservoir at or below heart level.

6. PATIENT CONNECTION

Although we prefer to use a dedicated cannula, PCA devices are commonly connected to the sidearm of an intravenous infusion which is supplying the patient's fluid requirements. It is important that the patient is protected from the possibility of drug backing up into the infusion set should the IV cannula be obstructed (Fig. 8.1 a–c). Temporary occlusion with immediate clearing would merely

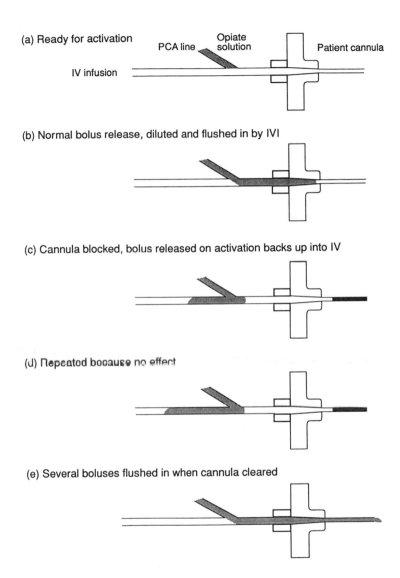

(a) Ready for activation

PCA line Opiate solution Patient cannula

IV infusion

(b) Normal bolus release, diluted and flushed in by IVI

(c) Cannula blocked, bolus released on activation backs up into IV

(d) Repeated because no effect

(e) Several boluses flushed in when cannula cleared

Fig. 8.1. Effect of blocked cannula with simple connection of PCA line to IVI line.

result in a slight delay in dose onset, but any prolonged obstruction would be likely to result in repeated demands because of the lack of effect, with the consequent danger of large amounts (the sum of several bolus doses) of drug running in if the obstruction is cleared without disconnection (Fig. 8.1 d–e). It is therefore mandatory to interpose a one-way (anti-reflux) valve with suitable design characteristics (Fig. 8.2). It is also vital that the PCA and infusion are connected to the correct ports of the one-way valve; if only one route is protected by a one-way valve, misconnection has led to backing up, with subsequent respiratory depression (Notcutt and Morgan 1990), although in this reported incident it was not sufficiently serious to warrant specific treatment. One-way valves must be clearly marked; it would be best if it were not possible to misconnect them, and this can be achieved by having one-way valves on both arms (see Chapter 6 for a further discussion of one-way valve design).

The lockout interval is designed to allow sufficient time for the major part of the bolus dose effects (both analgesic and respiratory) to be apparent. It is usually based on received wisdom regarding how long it takes for an intravenous injection of the particular drug to act. This tends to ignore possible delays between the PCA device and the patient's circulation due to the deadspace in the connections, which will be cleared at a rate depending on the rate of the IV infusion. It is therefore important to connect the one-way valve directly to the IV cannula so that a minimum of the lockout period is used up in this way: a large volume connector with a three-way tap, for instance, could nullify a short lockout if combined with a slow drip rate (Fig. 8.3). The use of a dedicated cannula for the PCA avoids both this hazard and the necessity for an anti-reflux valve, but this advantage unfortunately cannot be entirely guaranteed, since the cannula may be treated as a convenient replacement for a failed infusion cannula: staff unfamiliar with the requirements for PCA may then arrange a non-valved connection. Thorough taping and labelling is the best defence, since even the most comprehensive education programme will not reach all locum or agency staff; it should also prevent the use of the cannula for other intravenous medication, which may be incompatible with the narcotic solution.

Care must also be taken with priming tubing and one-way valves before connection to the patient. If drug solution is allowed to

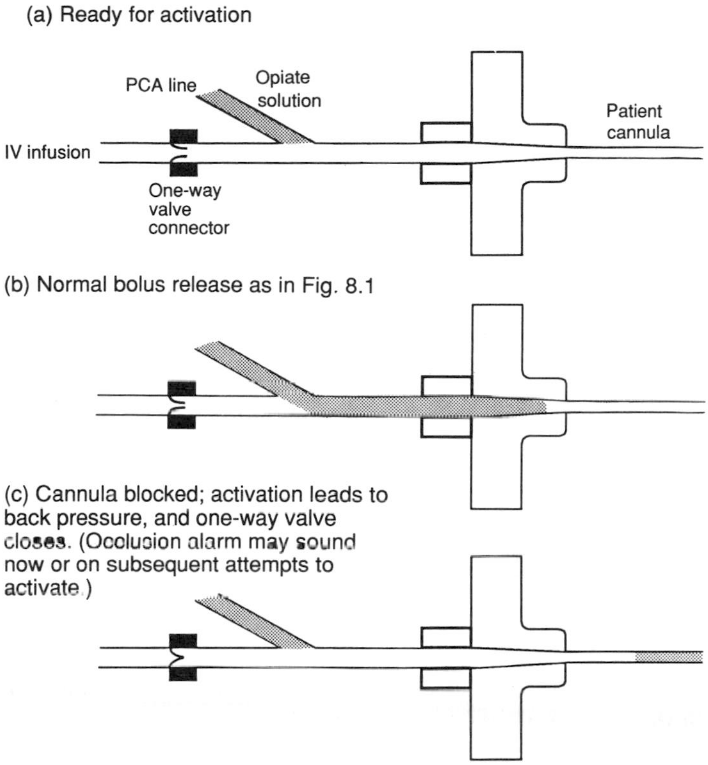

(a) Ready for activation

PCA line
Opiate solution
Patient cannula
IV infusion
One-way valve connector

(b) Normal bolus release as in Fig. 8.1

(c) Cannula blocked; activation leads to back pressure, and one-way valve closes. (Occlusion alarm may sound now or on subsequent attempts to activate.)

Fig. 8.2. One-way valve on IV line to present backing-up.

fill the valve, which is then connected to the patient without flushing, starting the infusion will deliver this internal volume to the patient without activation of the patient-demand switch (Fig. 8.4a and b). This is most unlikely to be hazardous, but may, by summation with the first dose, lead to overestimation of the effectiveness of the chosen bolus size. It is another reason for advocating relatively low drug concentrations; but the main safeguard is to specify that, after priming, the assembled system is flushed through with the infusion fluid before connecting to the patient (Fig. 8.4c).

Migration of the IV cannula outside the vein ('tissueing') can lead to bolus doses' being deposited subcutaneously. Because absorption

Patient-controlled analgesia

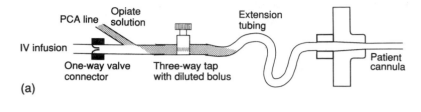

(a)

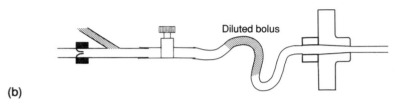

(b)

Fig. 8.3. Effect of extra deadspace: (a) normal bolus release; (b) slow progress of bolus with slow IV infusion rate—may take most of lockout period.

will be delayed analgesia will be reduced, and repeated demands may be made, leading to the possibility of depot formation and subsequent excessive absorption. This accident is more likely with dedicated cannulae, and with low-volume/high-concentration bolus doses. Choice of superficial veins, good supervision, instructing the patient to report changes in effectiveness, and the use of relatively high-volume bolus doses will all reduce this danger.

In practice, the majority of the problems listed above under headings 2–6 have not been reported to have endangered patients and are largely avoidable if clear protocols are followed; they will be minimized if the anaesthetist who has cared for the patient throughout the perioperative period not only orders the PCA regime but personally carries out the preparation and connection of the system and is available for consulation during the initial period of use.

7. ABNORMAL DRUG REACTIONS

True sensitivity to narcotic drugs is relatively rare, although morphine causes direct histamine release. Pethidine administered to patients on monoamine oxidase inhibitors can cause serious reactions; but we do not regard it as suitable for PCA for other reasons (see Chapter 3). Although anaphylaxis can occur after minute quantities of drugs, in general the relatively small doses of drugs used for PCA make all other types of reaction less likely to endanger the patient than conventional therapy; for other reasons, we have stressed the advantages of using the same drug intra- and postoperatively, and this virtually eliminates idiosyncracy as a postoperative hazard.

Adverse reactions to drugs should be reported via the well-established yellow card system. Where a defect of manufacture or processing is suspected it should be reported to the Department of Health (see the appendix to this chapter).

(a) One-way connector primed with opiate from PCA system

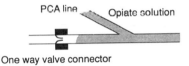

(b) Unrecorded dose flushed in on connection to patient

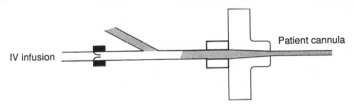

(c) Correct sequence: flush with IV fluid before connecting

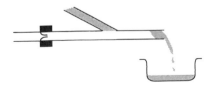

Fig. 8.4. Priming error.

8. EQUIPMENT MALFUNCTION

The sophisticated design of current models of electronic pumps includes internal self-checking procedures which, in the event of malfunction, lead the equipment to 'fail safe'—that is, no drug will be delivered and, normally, an alarm will sound. Nevertheless, accidents have occurred, and probably cannot be entirely avoided, as a result of equipment malfunction. This can result from poor design (Grover and Heath 1992) or from unforeseen interactions such as power surges (Health Departments SAB(90)85 1990; Notcutt *et al.* 1992). The incidence of accidents and related problems is discussed in Chapters 6 and 7. The procedures for reporting incidents are given in the appendix to this chapter. At the end of this book, readers will find an outline of the emergency treatment of respiratory depression due to opiate overdosage: 'Quick Guide 3'.

9. MOVING THE PATIENT AND THE EQUIPMENT

Most of the problems associated with moving the patient and/or the equipment do not endanger the patient, although they may well interfere with therapy or cause equipment damage. Probably the most dangerous possibility is that of failure to transmit full information about monitoring requirements and whom to contact if problems or emergencies arise. Badly designed activation switches can give an unintended bolus if dropped on the floor; however, little harm is likely from a single extra dose. Arcing is avoided if wall switches are switched off before equipment is unplugged; power surges from this cause and from static accumulation transmitted via the infusion pole have resulted in deprogramming or even overinfusion; but these faults should have been eliminated by modification of existing equipment and by redesign of current models.

10. ACTIVATION OF THE SYSTEM BY ANYONE OTHER THAN THE PATIENT

The crucial safety mechanism of PCA relies on the inability of a sedated or sleeping patient to make a demand. Any other person activating the switch in this situation is clearly capable of administering an unwanted dose. This can be done intentionally or unintentionally. The latter situation might arise if a nurse or visitor, perceiving an emergency, mistook the PCA demand switch for a nurse-call system button and used it in order to summon assistance. For this reason we favour an activation switch that is attached to the patient and does not resemble a nurse-call button. All staff need to be familiar with the equipment, and it should also be explained to patients' visitors. The size of the normal bolus dose makes it unlikely that a single extra dose would cause significant danger. There is significant danger if failure to understand PCA leads to nurses or patients' relatives deliberately activating the system. The duty anaesthetist in our hospital was called to see a patient who had become difficult to rouse and mildly respiratorily depressed whilst attached to PCA. No fault was detected in the equipment or prescription; but questioning the patient's wife revealed that she had interpreted snoring when he fell asleep as grunts of pain, and had therefore 'helped' by pressing the button. No treatment was needed, but a lesson was learned. Relatives (and nurses) must be specifically prohibited from pressing the button for the patient except in circumstances where the patient requires this physical assistance, and has clearly expressed the desire for a bolus. Units which involve parents in PCA for small children need to take particular care that there is real understanding of the system and close supervision.

11. LONG-TERM USE

It has often been stated that the addictive potential of narcotics can pose a risk to normal postoperative patients. We know of no good evidence to support this: the recent report from the Working Party on Acute Pain (The Royal College of Surgeons and the College of Anaesthetists 1990) extrapolated a possible figure of 1 in 3000 (derived from a study of the records of 11 000 medical patients in the USA (Porter and Jick 1979)) as an acceptable addiction risk for postoperative patients. This figure would be totally unacceptable to us, implying that our hospital might be generating two or three addicts per year from its surgical population. The experience of local psychiatrists responsible for addiction services accord with our view that the risk is almost non-existent. It is most unfortunate that the idea has been a major obstruction to the adequate treatment of postoperative pain. Current or recent intravenous drug abusers are clearly in a different category from the normal surgical population, and would best be treated by techniques relying on local anaesthetics. We would not use PCA for these patients unless there was some exceptional indication, and very close supervision would be required.

APPENDIX: REPORTING PROBLEMS WITH DRUGS OR EQUIPMENT

Reporting adverse drug reactions

All SERIOUS suspected reactions should be reported even if well recognized. NEW drugs (marked with black triangle in BNF, MIMS, and Data Sheets) should have ALL suspected reactions reported. YELLOW CARDS CAN BE FOUND IN MIMS & BNF AND ARE KEPT BY ALL HOSPITAL PHARMACIES. (There is a specially designed Yellow Card for anaesthetic reactions.)

Reporting defects in medicinal products

If you suspect a defect either in manufacture or processing of a drug you should contact:

> Defect Report Centre
> Medicines Control Agency
> Room 1801 Market Towers
> 1 Nine Elms Lane SW8 5NQ   Tel. 071 627 1513

Reporting equipment problems: National Reporting and Investigation Centre—NATRIC

This section of the Department of Health's Medical Devices Directorate (MDD) investigates:

- any safety-related incident or potentially harmful product/material, whether identified as such before use, during use, or as a result of an accident;

● problems arising through incorrect use of or inappropriate modification, adjustment, or maintenance of equipment, products, or materials; and

● minor incidents or anomalies which may be indicators of inadequate quality assurance on the part of the manufacturer or supplier.

A database of all reports and investigations is maintained.

HOW TO CONTACT NATRIC:
'HOT LINE' during normal office hours: 071 636 6811, ext. 3030
24-hour answering machine service: 071 637 1674
FAX number: 071 436 6764; BT Gold computer link: NHS 217.

Full written reports (purpose-designed forms are available) should follow as soon as possible to:

> Room 413
> Department of Health
> 14 Russell Square WC1B 5EP

In Wales, contact: Welsh Office
Health Services Planning Division
Cathays Park
Cardiff CF1 3NQ   Tel. 0222 823641

In Scotland: Scottish Health Service,
CSA Supplies Division
Trinity Park House
South Trinity Road
Edinburgh EH5 3SH Tel.: 031 552 6255 ext 2056

In N. Ireland: Department of Health and Social Services
Defect Centre
Estate Services Directorate
Stoney Road
Dundonald
Belfast BT16 OUS   Tel.: 0232 484535

Any equipment involved in a serious incident must be retained for inspection. A *Safety Action Bulletin* No. 63 (SAB (90) 61) issued jointly by the Health Departments outlines procedures and lists relevant Circulars.

If an event appears to be so serious that immediate action to protect patients is required outside office hours the Department of Health have a duty officer on call at Richmond House who can deal with such problems: call 071 210 5371/5368.

9 *Putting the equipment into use*

INTRODUCTION

The resource implications of PCA will be discussed in Chapter 10; in this chapter we assume that approval for the service has been obtained and the source of funding has been identified. The selection of equipment must take into account the matching of user requirements against the design factors discussed in Chapter 6. In addition, however, there are some non-patient-related factors to be considered. Once purchased, it is important that acceptance and commissioning are correctly carried out to ensure that the equipment arrives in the user department and can be safely put into service. Education of all staff groups who will come into contact with PCA equipment and/or care for patients using it is vital. There must be clear delineation of responsibilities for prescribing drug regimes for patients, programming electronic pumps, and dealing with untoward events. Matters pertaining to patient care and supervision will be dealt with in the Chapter 11; but the particular area of handover of responsibility, whether or not it involves movement of the patient and equipment between locations, merits special consideration. Finally, we revert to the basics of equipment management, to ensure that pumps are cared for properly and achieve maximum availability.

Box 19. Steps in the introduction of PCA equipment

1. Selection, acceptance, and commissioning
2. Staff education
3. Prescribing
4. Filling drug reservoirs
5. Programming and connection to patient
6. Transfer of supervision
7. Recharging of drug reservoirs
8. Storage, maintenance, and repair

---

1. SELECTION, ACCEPTANCE, AND COMMISSIONING

All hospitals must have departments responsible for the supervision of patient-related equipment, most of which has electronic components. These departments are variously named (Electronics, Electronic and Biomedical Equipment (EBME), Medical Equipment, etc.), and may be subdivisions of Works/Engineering or Medical Physics Departments; we will use EBME as a convenient abbreviation. It is worth understanding the structure in your own hospital because it determines, amongst other things, the hierarchy of communication (or lack of it) within the organization. This is especially important with regard to receipt of vital information such as Hazard Warnings, *Safety Information Bulletins*, and *Health Equipment Information* (the official NHS journal for disseminating evaluation reports and related advice). Just as crucial are the people and procedures (often in that order) involved in ordering and ensuring delivery of equipment and replacement parts.

It is common to accept equipment on loan from the supplier for trial purposes, and this is a good way of ensuring that the theoretical virtues, extolled persuasively by sales representatives, translate into the practical values of ease of use and staff acceptance. We cannot emphasize too strongly that all the advice that follows regarding acceptance and commissioning procedures (with appropriate modification) applies equally to loaned equipment. Disasters have been attributable to failure to follow this advice (Heath 1992).

The Senior Officer in EBME must be involved in the selection of the equipment, so that the level of in-house maintenance for which the pump is suitable can be identified and agreed. Clearly, the more that can be done without sending the equipment back to the supplier or arranging a special visit the better. Availability of replacement parts and full documentation are mandatory, and the track record of manufacturers and suppliers in terms of speed of response and helpfulness with advice are factors which should not be underestimated. Equipment lying unused, for whatever reason, is, in effect, a drain on resources, since only when it is in use can it supply the benefit end of the cost-benefit ratio.

Having selected the equipment desired, personal pressure may be required to smooth the passage of the order and minimize delivery delays; we have found no substitute for dogged, polite persistence.

Equipment must be delivered to EBME, never to the user department, so that it and its documentation can be thoroughly checked, marked, and added to the hospital equipment inventory. At this stage any training sessions needed for defined groups of staff should be arranged and a formal record should be made of attendance. Pumps currently available on the market have reached a high level of intrinsic safety, and probably more danger lies in the retention of older equipment, especially since it is likely to be used less frequently. Those in charge of PCA therapy should review the need for refresher training and for withdrawing from use infrequently used equipment, or at least for labelling it to draw the attention of users to the need to seek advice from those familiar with it.

2. STAFF EDUCATION

Although this chapter is primarily devoted to the practicalities of using the equipment, we feel that the importance of staff education cannot be repeated too often. As well as a programme of initial instruction in use of the equipment, which will primarily be directed towards anaesthetists and Recovery Room staff, it is vital to ensure that all staff caring for patients understand the principles of PCA. Small tutorials seem to be the best method, backed up by one-to-one practical teaching at all the different stages of care. No one should underestimate the amount of effort and persistence that has to be put into this aspect: misunderstandings creep in with amazing frequency. An open offer to repeat training sessions whenever needed makes education a two-way process, as the instructor will learn from the varied experience of staff. Clearly, staff dedicated to an Acute Pain Team will be best placed to be effective. It may be difficult to ensure participation of all staff, even at the start, and it is therefore important to identify key people who can activate a cascade of training. Being able to do something, particularly something which has safety considerations, is not the same as being able to teach someone else to do it—a vital check may be carried out so swiftly that it is not obvious unless made explicit—and the ability to supervise and correct mistakes patiently (rather than to lean over and do the job) is not given to everyone. Anaesthetists and nurses are the commonest groups from which such trainers will be drawn, but personality characteristics will be of most importance in determining their effectiveness; enthusiasm and persistence are necessary supplements to knowledge.

3. PRESCRIBING THE REGIME

The most appropriate person to prescribe the PCA regime is the anaesthetist, whose care of the patient starts preoperatively. Assessment of the patients' physical and psychological states will determine their preoperative treatment, and the effects of premedication and anaesthetic technique and the response to operative trauma will all allow a better judgement of the initial prescription for postoperative pain relief. It is mainly for these reasons we would not favour handing over responsibility to an Acute Pain Team until after the immediate recovery period. In addition, we feel that all anaesthetists should become familiar with PCA both in theory and practice, and this is best ensured by thinking of the initial prescription and assessment as the final part of the anaesthetic technique. Safe, easy prescribing is aided by a purpose-designed form, since few standard prescription charts allow the identification of all the necessary information. We have designed a form that will stick on to the Lewisham Hospital chart (see appendix to this chapter). Although standardization between hospitals is desirable, the evolution of a suitable chart is an educational exercise that can aid the understanding and involvement of medical, nursing, and pharmacy staff with advantage. The basic information needed in addition to patient identification consists of:

(a) the equipment to be used
    (name of electronic pump or disposable device);
(b) total drug, dilution volume, and consequent concentration
    (for initial and each subsequent charging);
(c) the bolus dose and lockout interval chosen
    (with spaces for up to three revisions);
(d) intravenous site, and whether dedicated or with one-way valve;

(e) date and time of commencement and termination of therapy;

(f) volume of solution (and consequent mass of drug) disposed of at end of therapy; and

(g) calculated total dose received by patient.

Each line for item (c) requires space for the full signature of the prescribing doctor, and each line for (b) requires space for clear initials identifying both the person charging the device and the person checking the procedure. Item (f) requires spaces for initials identifying the disposer and the checker.

In our view there is convincing evidence (discussed in Chapter 3) that background infusions do not, in general, enhance efficacy or safety; we have therefore elected for simplicity, and made no explicit provision for their prescription, although there is space in which such variations from the norm could be specified if required. A reminder to prescribe antiemetic drugs (on the routine chart) is also helpful.

When PCA therapy is being established within a hospital there is much to be said in favour of a standard protocol which lessens the number of choices facing the prescriber at a time when familiarization with the equipment and setting-up procedure need to be the first priority: acceptance of a new treatment is much more likely if complexity is reduced as far as possible. The basis for choosing the appropriate drug, bolus dose, and lockout period have been discussed in Chapter 3. We have found papaveretum 2 mg/ml and a 2 mg bolus with a lockout of 6 minutes a satisfactory basic regime. Following advice issued by the Committee on Safety of Medicines which precludes the use of this drug in females of child-bearing potential, we use morphine in this group. Other centres have used diamorphine (Notcutt and Morgan 1990) or morphine (Wheatley *et al.* 1991) (both 1 mg/ml) with success. If it is decided initially to suggest a standard bolus dose there should be a plan to encourage individualized prescribing as soon as possible, so that patients can obtain adequate pain relief without either very frequent button-pressing (for those with high drug requirements), or excessive side-effects (in those whose needs are much lower). Review soon after starting therapy, as is advocated in Chapter 11, is the key to optimizing the regime; however, it must be borne in mind that the fixed bolus volume of the disposable device limits flexibility.

4. FILLING THE DRUG RESERVOIR

Charging of syringes or disposable devices may be carried out by pharmacy staff, although this involves prior selection of the drug concentration, without the knowledge afforded during the operative procedure. This is unlikely to be a disadvantage with programmable pumps, since bolus dose and lockout interval need not be selected until therapy is about to be started; however, the only currently available disposable device has a fixed bolus volume and lockout interval, and therefore selection of drug concentration is the only way in which the bolus dose can be altered. Nevertheless, this use of pharmacy staff may be regarded as a safe and convenient aid for the busy anaesthetist, although it involves a certain amount of extra bother for other staff, who must ensure transfer of the prescription chart to the pharmacy and delivery of the charged syringe or device to the recovery room, where it will need to be stored in the controlled drugs cupboard. It makes the provision of a separate PCA prescription chart highly desirable, since the chart will be absent from the ward for a substantial period. Where large numbers of patients are being treated and sterile preparation facilities exist in the pharmacy, it may be possible to keep stocks of ready-prepared syringes within the Recovery Room. Syringes will need to be kept in a controlled drugs refrigerator with appropriate security. Normal procedures can then be followed for issuing and recording syringes for individual patients. Full labelling, including date of preparation and date beyond which a syringe should be discarded if unused, will be required. Unless there is a relatively high and steady level of demand, such a system may prove wasteful.

It may be felt that recovery room nursing staff are sufficiently familiar with the drugs used to allow them to take on the responsibility of filling the drug reservoir according to the prescription. We would not recommend this, because of the crucial importance of obtaining the correct drug concentration, as discussed in Chapter 8. There is usually a convenient time towards the end of the operation or shortly after transfer to the recovery room when the anaesthetist can prepare the drug solution, with the anaesthetic assistant or a recovery room nurse checking the procedure. A busy period in the recovery room can preclude releasing two appropriately trained staff simultaneously, and so it seems best for the anaesthetist to take the prime responsibility. Similar considerations apply on ordinary postoperative wards, where ensuring appropriate training for enough staff is likely to be difficult and inefficient; in addition, any significant overdose resulting from an error will be less easily noticed and treated than in a recovery room. The development of High-Dependency Units for postoperative patients should provide a more appropriate setting for nurses to take over recharging syringes, as will Intensive Therapy Units if PCA becomes more commonly used within them. It is good practice to attach a self-adhesive label indicating the drug, dilution, and personnel involved. The label must not obscure the syringe markings, and when the syringe is loaded into the pump, the graduations need to be visible with the cover closed, so that consumption can be monitored and the volume of solution remaining when therapy is stopped can be read off easily.

5. PROGRAMMING AND CONNECTING THE EQUIPMENT

The start of PCA therapy using an electronic pump involves programming in addition to charging with drug solution. The responsibility for programming rests with the prescribing doctor, and again we see strong practical and theoretical reasons for this being the patient's anaesthetist. Whilst user-friendly, logical prompts are now a feature of modern pump design, it is essential to have the manufacturer's instructions immediately available and to refer to them during training sessions. Standardization of equipment minimizes the chances of error, particularly with regard to choice of disposables. A second, trained person who understands fully the basis of PCA and is familiar with, as well as being technically able to be responsible for, the opiate drugs should always check each stage.

Many pumps incorporate a priming facility: this is best ignored, since inadvertent selection of this option after connecting to the patient could be an all-too-simple recipe for overinfusion. Despite various built-in safeguards and warnings we fear the unfathomable ingenuity of the inspired meddler. Manual priming of the connecting line away from the patient remains the safer choice. Similarly, the loading-dose option present on some pumps is a needless complication. Patients whose intraoperative analgesia proves to have been inadequate are best treated by direct titration using a separate syringe of the chosen opiate. Increments of twice to two and a half times the anticipated bolus dose are suitable. It is not uncommon to require quite large doses in total (10–20 mg morphine) at this stage, and it is clearly foolish to try to guess an appropriate single large dose.

Direct connection of the line to a dedicated cannula is the simplest and safest scheme, and one that we would recommend as a routine. Choose a site that will be most convenient for the patient and nursing staff, bearing in mind that pain relief may be desirable after discontinuation of intravenous fluid therapy. The deliberate choice of a small-gauge cannula should discourage its being 'borrowed' for IV fluid if the original drip fails: we have found a patient whose PCA cannula had been reconnected for this purpose using only a three-way tap: the absence of a one-way valve constituting an obvious hazard. However, cannulae with high intrinsic resistance, such as the Y-can, which has a very-narrow-bore sidearm, should not be used, since they are likely to generate high pressures during bolus administration, and thus activate the occlusion alarm even though they are patent; this is both puzzling and infuriating for staff. The cannula and connection should be secured in such a way that extravasation has the best possible chance of becoming immediately apparent; and we also recommend labelling the site to prohibit unauthorized rearrangement.

If the PCA line is connected as a side-channel to an IV infusion it is imperative that a Y-connector incorporating a one-way valve on the IV arm is used to avoid opiate backing up into the drip should the cannula block (see Figs. 8.1 and 8.2, pp. 107, 109).

The advantages of connecting PCA as a side-channel to an IV infusion lie in the more rapid recognition of extravasation and fewer problems with blocked cannulae. Disadvantages (discussed in Chapters 6 and 8) include the extra deadspace of a one-way valve; the greater care needed in priming the system (drug solution must enter the main channel and then be flushed through with the IV solution to ensure an accurate first dose, but no 'extra' from the prime: see Fig. 8.4, p.111; the possibility of stored volume during temporary occlusion; and the possibility of malfunction or misconnection. They are also relatively expensive (see Chapter 10). If a Y-connector is used we would favour a pattern that has one-way valves on both arms, and therefore cannot be misconnected. We have not, however, found one that is available, and it therefore remains important that everyone understands precisely what the function is, since they are then more likely to connect it correctly.

Completion of connection should be marked by checking that the relevant sections of the prescription chart have been filled in, signed, or initialled. The supervision of the equipment is then handed over to the person responsible for looking after the patient—normally the recovery room nurse.

6. TRANSFER OF SUPERVISION

Handover of patient care between nursing staff requires transfer of responsibility for the particular PCA equipment in use: this entails ensuring that the new carer understands how it works, and the principles of PCA therapy as well as the nursing requirements. The details of the prescription should be checked, together with the name and bleep number of the on-site doctor who is to be contacted in case of problems—this will usually be one of the duty anaesthetists; in addition, we have found it reassuring for staff if the home telephone number of an appropriate consultant anaesthetist is added. We have also attached to each pump copies of the information sheets for patients and staff (see appendix to Chapter 5)

If the patient is being moved a record should be made of his or her name, hospital number, and destination within the hospital, together with the date and time of transfer and the identification details for the pump. This allows easy tracking of equipment, identification of patients currently on PCA therapy, and simple audit of this aspect of postoperative pain relief. A standard hospital diary is cheap and easily adapted for this purpose, and will form a permanent, durable record. In addition, an equipment-location board is extremely useful for the rapid identification both of patients currently on PCA and of available pumps. Pumps do not require to be switched off during transfer—all modern mains-operated equipment has battery back-up—but it is good practice to switch off the wall socket before disconnecting a mains plug; earlier designs were susceptible to program loss because of power surges, but this fault is said to have been corrected by the provision of new software for existing equipment and eliminated during the design of current models. Security features, which include key-operated clamping to the drip-stand, tend to be a nuisance and therefore self-defeating. If the pump cannot be secured to the trolley rail it may be laid on the trolley or bed during transfer; but care should be taken that connecting line and the patient's activating pendant are not tangled or damaged. Locating the drug reservoir no higher than the level of the patient's heart at all times will effectively eliminate the possibility of drug solution syphoning into the patient should an accident favour this. Currently available pumps using plastic syringes have an extremely low potential for syphonage, and the Baxter disposable device cannot syphon.

7. RECHARGING THE DRUG RESERVOIR

Trained nurses dedicated to the Acute Pain Team are probably the ideal persons to undertake recharging of drug reservoirs by preparing fresh syringes or fitting replacement syringes prepared by Pharmacy. In the absence of a full Acute Pain Team we currently feel that responsibility for recharging and reconnecting the drug reservoir should remain with anaesthetic staff, the procedure being checked by a second person in exactly the same way as for the initial preparation. It is possible that pharmacy staff could prepare drug solutions and suitably trained ward nurses could exchange syringes; however, this increases the number of people involved in calculation and checking; it could produce documentation problems; and it will probably remain inadvisable on ordinary wards, certainly until the use of PCA has become so widespread that virtually all staff are familiar with its principles and practice. Hospitals with stable nurse staffing have found that it is possible to train sufficient numbers of nurses to assign syringe-changing to the ward staff. This normally means that a rigid system of a single drug used at a fixed dilution must be imposed, and requires the total co-operation of all members of the anaesthetic department. Whilst the latter factor is not a major problem, staff turnover in our hospital (as explained elsewhere) has thwarted our efforts to maintain a PCA-trained nurse on every ward at all times. We have also had continual turbulence in terms of the allocation of types of surgical work to particular wards. Colleagues in other inner-city hospitals confirm that this is common; and the future holds major reorganization for the whole of London at the very least.

Electronic pumps often have a 'syringe nearly empty' warning, so that therapy is not interrupted by delay in recharging. We do not advise relying on this, however, since it is quite easy to assess the individual consumption rate after a few hours of treatment and therefore to predict the most convenient time for recharging (see Box 20). It is the one situation where calculations in volume (rather than mass) units seem more sensible.

Box 20. Example of calculation of consumption and prediction of syringe emptying time

Volume of reservoir   = 60 ml
Time PCA commenced   = 15.30
Time of assessment   = 18.30
Volume remaining in syringe = 48 ml
Therefore consumption   = 12 ml in 3 hr or 4ml/hr

The remaining 48 ml will last 48/4 = 12 hrs, and syringe may empty before 06.30 tomorrow morning. Suggest refilling any convenient time after 19.00, since full syringe = 15 hr and will then last till 10.00.

Also consider increasing drug concentration and bolus dose for this relatively high user.

Ensuring recharging at sensible times is one of the functions of the evening round described in Chapter 11. Disturbance during normal sleeping time is bad for patients, their neighbours, and the anaesthetist who has to perform the task. The procedure for replenishing the reservoir will vary with the equipment being used; it is therefore important that the instructions are readily available, so that the operator does not have to rely on memory. The solution must be prepared and checked against the prescription, and both chart and controlled drug records completed. The local protocol should take account of both the model of pump and the type of connecting lines in use, since these affect the possibility of accidental infusion of extra solution by pressure on the syringe plunger, particularly whilst it is being inserted into the drive mechanism. Soft-walled lines can be clamped to prevent this possibility, but care must be taken to ensure that the clamp is released at the end of the procedure. Accidental occlusion at other times may be more likely with these connecting lines. If non-kinking lines are used, disconnection of the system during recharging will prevent inadvertent drug administration; but we do not recommend this—contamination or even misconnection become a possibility. We feel that it is sufficient to stress that the person changing the syringe must take care not to press on the syringe plunger. So long as our advice to use relatively weak solutions of drugs (leading to bolus doses of more than 0.5 ml) is followed, the chance of significant overdosage during syringe-changing seems remote.

8. STORAGE, MAINTENANCE, AND REPAIR

Postoperative wards are often keen to own their own equipment, and frequently fund-raise to supplement inadequate budgets. Whilst the enthusiasm and involvement generated can be beneficial to patients and staff, and equipment may be better cared for by staff who 'own' it, there are distinct disadvantages to disseminating equipment. Matching patients in need to available pumps will inevitably lead to borrowing, and it is much better for the hospital stock of pumps to be kept in one place: the recovery room is clearly the best placed to oversee the equipment. Pumps should be returned to the recovery room as soon as is reasonably convenient after PCA is discontinued; if the stock of available pumps is low, the equipment location record makes it easy for the ward to be reminded of this. Good liaison with postoperative wards is essential to ensure that any problems are notified and that equipment is returned complete and clean.

The EBME department will be responsible for a regular maintenance programme, though this will not usually need to consist of much more than checking of leads and basic performance and alarms. Again this is made much easier if one place is 'home' for all the pumps. They will also keep a log of any repairs required and review the reliability and robustness of equipment. The experience gained from these functions forms the basis of the advice available from the EBME department when replacement or expansion of the equipment stock is undertaken; it sometimes happens that equipment with a low initial price leads to high running costs because of frequent breakdowns and expensive spare parts, although we curently know of no PCA equipment to which this applies.

APPENDIX: LEWISHAM HOSPITAL PCA PRESCRIPTION CHART

PATIENT LABEL/DETAILS

LEWISHAM HOSPITAL

Patient-Controlled Analgesia Prescription and Record Form

PCA system: (circle) Graseby 3300, Graseby PCAS, Cardiff Palliator, Baxter Infuser, Other....

IV Site: (circle) Right, Left, hand, forearm, other.......... (circle) Dedicated cannula/ via sidearm of one-way valve on infusion.

Date	Time	Prescription Drug	bolus mg	lockout min	quantity total mg	volume total ml	Diluent	corcn mg/ml	(bolus vol) (= ml)	prescriber	Syringe contents made up by	checked by

Antiemetics prescribed on main chart?

PCA discontinued at (time) _____ (date) _____ Volume remaining in syringe: _____ ml signed: _____ (ward nurse)

Total dose received by patient: _____ mg

Other information:

Any problems, contact Dr _____ or duty SHO Anaesthetics.

10   Resources and PCA

Health-care workers, and doctors in particular, have been accustomed to introducing new treatments purely on the basis of their perceived benefits. However, in a cash-limited service, extra money spent on a new activity has to be diverted from some other activity, and this has meant an increasing emphasis on cost-benefit analysis (Maynard 1987). At its simplest, this might be illustrated by the introduction of a new formulation of a drug that allowed, at the same daily drug cost, oral treatment instead of injections: therapeutic benefit identical, no change in side-effects, nicer for the patient, and the cost of needles and syringes saved; all the information points in a desirable direction. This simplicity unfortunately has the rarity of snow in summer: layers of complexity are added in most instances by the need to consider, on the benefit side, detractions and modifications (such as side-effects) and on the cost side, the need for additional monitoring, staff time, etc. Since the money in question can come from different budgets (for example hospital or GP drug budgets) and even different services (for example NHS or Social Services) the difficulty of the assessment is only matched by the difficulty of obtaining a decision for change.

It is tempting to question the cost-benefit ratio of the new industry that has taken off in response to this trend: we will resist that temptation and make a cautious attempt to review the resource implications of PCA. The other side of the equation—the balance of benefits—is dealt with in the remainder of the book, and readers may make their own judgements on the case.

THE COST FRAMEWORK

The easiest costs to grapple with are those associated with an individual patient; to these must be added an appropriate fraction of the overall costs of the whole service. It is clear that the more patients are treated, the more the first element will rise, but the smaller the fraction per patient of whole-service costs incurred. We can make no pretence to any great accuracy in our costings, which are based on 1991 contract prices (where appropriate). In the box we list the elements to be considered, and have used the standard 'financial' coding convention whereby items that are saved from the intramuscular injection (IMI) regime are indicated in brackets.

Box 21. The financial equation: each case

| COSTS PER PATIENT FOR PCA | (SAVINGS FROM IMI) |

disposables: cannula or connector,
syringe, line,   (syringes)
PCA infuser—if chosen

drug and diluent   (drug)
staff time: preop information
equipment set-up
recovery initiation   (IMI in recovery)
ward supervision   (IMIs in ward)
                                  (hospital 'hotel' costs)

Whole-service costs consist of the outlay on pumps and their maintenance plus the cost of any staff time dedicated to the PCA service (as opposed to patient-care). The box shows them divided conventionally into capital and revenue.

Box 22. The financial equation: the PCA service

WHOLE-SERVICE COSTS
CAPITAL   REVENUE

PCA pumps   equipment: maintenance
            staff: Acute Pain Team

The capital costs are solely those of purchasing computerized PCA machines, and will be eliminated if it is decided to run the service entirely on the disposable, single-patient device (the Baxter Infuser).

[In the recently reorganized NHS, equipment costing more than £1000 is placed on a capital asset register (Working Paper 5, NHS Review 1989), and hospitals are required to make a 6 per cent return annually on this value. Allowance is therefore made for this factor in the prices charged to purchasing authorities, which in turn receive funding intended to account for this element. It is not yet known how (or even if) this system will influence decision-making, and for this reason, and because the amount in relation to PCA per patient would be extremely small, we propose to ignore it.]

OPPORTUNITY COSTS

Examination of the items listed under individual patient costs reveals that many are opportunity costs rather than money spent: staff who are employed for a given period of time may have to omit something that they now do in order to give time to PCA-related work. Patients are routinely assessed preoperatively and given information by ward and anaesthetic staff; modifying that process to include PCA-related matters may not increase time spent if postoperative pain relief is already being discussed. Time spent by anaesthetists in charging syringes, programming pumps, and inserting additional cannulae may be fitted into relatively quiescent periods of anaesthetic management, but on occasion will undoubtedly add a few minutes to turn-round time during a list. It can be more efficient for pharmacists to prepare drug reservoirs (syringes or infusers) in batches with a standard drug and concentration. The time taken will nevertheless be about ten minutes per patient (Taylor and Heath 1992). Similarly, ward supervision takes time, but may be undertaken by staff whose work programme has some slack in it at the appropriate time. Set against this is the genuine saving in nurse time spent in giving individual injections (each of which requires additional checking). In our hospital, experienced nurses were asked how long it took to perform safety checks on patients receiving PCA and how long to administer IM injections to patients on a prn regime. The assessment showed that on average, 42 minutes of nursing time were saved in the first 24 hours postoperatively if the patient received PCA rather than IM injections prn (Thomas *et al.* 1990). It is particularly important to note that the time that is eliminated is mainly time spent away from the patient, and that it is necessarily nursing time at the highest ward skill level. Financial, social, and demographic pressures are all combining to stress the provision of sufficient skilled nurses; it is therefore particularly valuable to reduce what is essentially a wastage of their time. Even the disposables do not increase total costs by their full amount, since they replace the syringe and needle costs of individual IM injections; there will, however, be an element of drug wastage, since large quantities are drawn up to allow for patients who have a high rate of uptake, and low users will only consume a small amount. Some approximate costings have been ascribed to the 'real money' elements and are set out in below.

Box 23. Comparison of costs of consumables

PCA patient:

cannula	30p (or one-way connector £2)
50 ml syringe	60p
line	30p
papaveretum 120 mg	78p
saline 3×20 ml	18p
Total:	£2.16–£3.86

IMI patient: average: 4 injections of 20 mg papaveretum.

4×2 ml syringes	24p
80 mg papaveretum	52p
Total:	76p

Net additional cost per PCA patient for consumables £1.40–£3.10.

If the service is run with disposable devices the additional cost per patient is simply the £16 per device (contract price). If programmable pumps are used (average cost approximately £2925, inc. VAT) it is necessary to assign a length of time over which this capital will be amortised, and therefore an annual charge on the service and to estimate the number of patients that it is likely to be used for. We have found a very low expenditure on spare parts for pumps, though this may tend to rise as they age, and we have allowed accordingly. Later in this chapter we will examine how to estimate the total number of pumps required; clearly, for a given surgical workload, the more pumps owned the higher the likelihood of a particular patient's being able to receive PCA, but the lower the number of patients each pump will be used on. It is worth making the best possible estimates when the decisions are made on the details of the service; here, however we are examining the overall case. For the moment we will assume an equipment life of

8 years, an average annual spare-part cost of £20, and an average use on 150 patients per year. This gives a cost per patient attributable to provision of programmable pumps of about £2.60. Thus it will be seen that additional costs for 'materials' range from £3.50 to £19 approximately. A policy of using dedicated cannulae, advocated on safety and efficacy grounds in Chapter 9, is also economical, since an additional cannula is cheaper than a one-way valve.

THE ACUTE PAIN TEAM

Real additional costs will be incurred if dedicated staff time is given to the Acute Pain Team. This usually takes the form of additional nursing hours, and is needed as much for teaching, trouble-shooting, and staff supervision as for individual patient-care. Units which have managed to institute such teams are in no doubt of their value. Without this backup, the chances of realizing the improvements possible and minimizing mismanagement are reduced. Our estimates are based on a part-time sister (20 hours of Grade G nursing time, total employment costs including London allowances £10 800), enabling an Acute Pain Service for 12 000 surgical cases per year, of which 1750 might receive PCA. The basis for this estimate is detailed later in this chapter. If the nursing contribution to other aspects of the Acute Pain Team's work is ignored and the total cost is ascribed to the PCA patients it will be seen that approximately £6 is added to the costs of each episode.

Allocation of one session per week of a consultant anaesthetist's time for overall supervision adds a further £2, leading to a grand total in the order of £12–£26. More generous provision of staff time can easily have cost estimates assigned.

SAVINGS GENERATED BY REDUCED LENGTH OF STAY

The final step in the assessment of the resource implications of the introduction of PCA as a substantial service requires consideration of the important findings on its effect on length of stay after major surgery. We have found no studies examining the effects of other pain-relief regimes as alternatives to the standard IMI prn. A study carried out in our hospital (Thomas 1991) has confirmed the finding of a significant reduction in length of postoperative stay (Clark *et al.* 1989) following major surgery. Sixty patients receiving PCA were compared with 64 having IMI following a variety of operations (abdominal hysterectomy, cholecystectomy, hip replacement, bowel surgery, oophorectomy); average length of stay postoperatively was 7.28 for PCA patients and 9.45 for IMI. Patients in this study received PCA only for the first 24 hours; one must be somewhat cautious, therefore, in extrapolating the findings to longer periods of use: longer seems most likely to be even better, but it could conceivably detract. Current estimates of 'hotel costs' on our wards suggest that, on average, the use of PCA, far from costing more, could save at least £150 per patient. To realize such savings requires either that more patients are treated (so that bed occupancy does not reduce), resulting in increased costs for theatre services, etc., or that in-patient accommodation is reorganized, with an overall reduction in staffed bed days. Wards may be closed completely, or some may be reduced to 5-day working. An estimate of the possibilities suggests that 1750 PCA patients could save 3500 bed-days, approximately equivalent to 10 beds—this is insufficient in itself to allow closure of a full ward, but may do so in combination with other measures, such as an increase in the proportion of procedures performed as day-cases. Further tentative support for cost-reduction is provided by the observation (Wheatley *et al.* 1990) that fewer chest infections were treated in general surgical patients in a year following introduction of the Acute Pain Service than in the year preceding it (0.4 per cent vs. 1.3 per cent of discharges); this service used PCA for approximately 6 per cent and epidural infusion analgesia for 2 per cent of cases, and further studies would be needed to determine the exact associations.

We would thus argue that resource estimates reinforce the clinical case for PCA rather than requiring difficult judgements—a June snow shower after all!

PRODUCING THE MOST ECONOMIC SERVICE

A small investment of time will allow decisions on the details of the service to be made with more confidence than mere guesswork. Some readers may have been surprised at the costings produced so far, and we hope that this will prompt them to pay some attention to details—carelessness in this area may not cost lives, but money disappears all too easily, with frustrating results.

Our estimate of the number of patients that one might expect to treat per PCA pump per year was made by surveying Recovery Room records for a period of 29 consecutive days to yield figures for the daily number of PCA patients that 28 days of normal operating workload might generate (Fig. 10.1). Each adult admission to the recovery room for a major general surgical, gynaecological, obstetric, or orthopaedic operation likely to require pain relief for 24 hours or more was noted. It was recognized that a number of patients included might be unsuitable (for example, because of mental impairment) and that some omitted (children, patients transferred direct to ITU, or those undergoing 'minor' but painful orthopaedic operations) might in reality be deemed suitable; the resultant inaccuracy should be relatively minor. Adding consecutive numbers for pairs of days yields the daily requirement for PCA pumps if each patient received PCA for about 48 hours for example, on Tuesday evening six patients would be receiving treatment if Monday's lists generated 4 and Tuesday's 2; by Wednesday evening 4 pumps would have returned to stock, but the total in operation might be 8 if that day's lists contained 4 suitable patients and 2 emergencies from the night had also been placed on pumps (Fig.

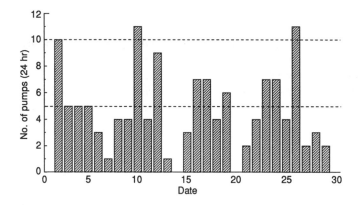

Fig. 10.1. Patients judged suitable for PCA during a 29-day period. On a basis of only 24 hours of treatment per patient, these figures therefore also represent the numbers of PCA pumps required per day.

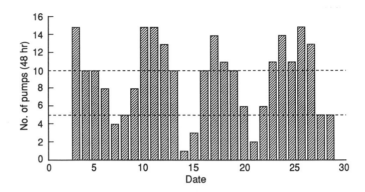

Fig. 10.2. Numbers of PCA pumps required per day to treat the same number of patients as in Fig. 10.1 on a basis of 48 hours of treatment per patient.

10.2) Multiplying the total by 13 to cover 52 weeks in the year allows an estimate of approximately 1750 PCA patients per year; the total surgical workload in our hospital (including day-cases) is approximately 12 000. Clearly, this intensity of usage will not be achieved initially, and reports on the introduction of PCA into two similar-sized district hospitals (Notcutt and Morgan 1990; Wheatley *et al.* 1991) imply that one-third of this rate will be reached in the initial years.

HOW MANY PUMPS TO HAVE AVAILABLE?

Considerable variation can be seen, the maximum being 15 (reached on four occasions), as seen in Fig. 10.2 and it is possible to examine the effects of various ways of providing a service. We have assumed that a pump will not be returned within less than 24 hours, and that all pumps will be returned within 48 hours. In practice, neither will be true; in particular, we have found that about 10 per cent of patients would like to continue PCA for more than 48 hours. It is reasonable to assume that these errors will roughly balance each other in the elective surgical population; however, increasing familiarity with the technique will certainly lead to prolonged usage in the occasional patient: the services at York and Great Yarmouth both record individual treatments in excess of 200 hours.

'LUXURY' PROVISION

Providing the maximum found to be required—fifteen—reduces the likely average number of patients treated per pump to 117, and this increases the cost per patient by less than £1. It is nevertheless inevitable that this amount of capital (nearly £44,000) will not be immediately available, and therefore the effects (costs incurred and benefits lost) of underprovision should be assessed.

EFFECTS OF HAVING FEWER PROGRAMMABLE PUMPS

Using the same survey data we may examine the different possibilities at two levels of underprovision: 10 and 5 pumps—illustrated by the horizontal lines on Figs. 10.1 and 10.2. Of the 135 patients thought likely to be suitable for PCA in the 4-week period we studied, only 93 (69 per cent) patients could have had 48 hours treatment with 10 pumps available, and 25 (19 per cent) with 5.

FIRST DAY ONLY

Restricting use to 24 hours (and ensuring prompt return of pumps) can increase the number benefiting from a smaller pump stock. Since pain is maximal during the the early postoperative hours, and many studies showing the advantages of PCA have been restricted to the first 24 hours, this is clearly a not unreasonable strategy. On this basis, in the time-period we studied, only 2 patients would have been denied PCA had 10 pumps been available; but the number rises to 29 for 5 pumps. These results are derived by counting the cases appearing above the two cut-off lines in Fig. 10.1.

Without denying more patients, a flexible strategy that allowed patients to keep the pump for 48 hours when possible would have allowed this length of treatment for 93 and 25 patients respectively; however, this would frequently entail difficult decisions about which patients should receive the longer treatment. Although intensive use of pumps is theoretically possible (perfect application of the flexible strategy would lead to 10 pumps serving 173 patients each per year and 5 serving 286), experience suggests that these levels are extremely unlikely to be achieved; hence we have proposed 150 patients per year as a reasonable target. These estimates make no allowance for 'downtime' (equipment out of service for maintenance or repair); but problems so far encountered have been minor and rapidly remedied.

'TOPPING UP' WITH THE DISPOSABLE DEVICE

Although relatively expensive, the disposable device (Baxter Infusor) has several advantages in particular circumstances (see Chapter 11). It may therefore be preferred for some patients, and can certainly be used to allow PCA for more patients when all programmable pumps are in use. The costs of using it at times of heaviest need can be examined.

The estimation has to consider each day sequentially, because the combinations of peaks and troughs of activity are also affected by the use of the disposable device, which serves a complete patient-treatment episode. To ensure 48-hour availability for all patients would have needed 26 units to supplement 10 pumps and 67 to supplement 5—noticeably less than appears at first sight, but nevertheless a substantial annual outlay of £5408 or £13,936 (subtract cost of 50 ml syringe and line from unit cost).

It is necessary to bear in mind the limitations of extrapolation; where more detailed information on the distribution of types of cases is sought, a six-week period has been judged necessary (Taylor *et al.* 1969).

TARGETTING PCA AT THOSE MOST HELPED

Despite our conviction that the case for comprehensive provision of PCA for postoperative pain relief is overwhelming, we recognize that not everyone will be instantly converted, nor can we ensure total availability speedily; many services will approach the regime with caution. Studies at Lewisham Hospital (described in Chapter 15) indicate that there is a very strong correlation between personality profiles and pain experience. Patients with high levels of state anxiety and coping styles that favour high levels of information-seeking and control will obtain the greatest reduction in pain scores as a result of using PCA. Where the ability to provide PCA is limited for whatever reason, targetting it to this type of patient will produce the maximal benefit. Studies are in progress to validate a simplified questionnaire that can be administered preoperatively to identify such patients with more certainty; meanwhile anaesthetists will do well to bear in mind that extra effort given to providing PCA for patients who obviously fall into these categories will be particularly well repaid.

11 Managing the patient and the regime

Early in this book we introduced the idea that reduction in the patient's sensitivity to pain could be considered at the very first contact. The importance of psychological factors should be held in mind throughout, and one should take care to assess the patient's personality and reaction to this particular set of circumstances (being in hospital for this operation with all its immediate and long-term implications). This sets the scene within which the choice of words both offering information and seeking the patient's reaction to it must be considered. All staff should have the same aim: to ensure that patients feel that their existence and experience are of the utmost importance.

During the treatment episode involving PCA, care of the patient changes in emphasis between nursing, surgical, anaesthetic, and other staff. In Box 24 we have tried to indicate which team member will predominate during each of the succeeding components that are most relevant to PCA.

Box 24. PCA 'lead worker' as hospital stay progresses

General information: ward nurse
    Specific information: anaesthetist
    intraoperative analgesia: anaesthetist
    appropriate prescription: anaesthetist
        first use/observations: recovery nurse
        initial assessment (and adjustment if necessary): recovery nurse/anaesthetist
            Ward observation: ward nurse
            encouragement/refinement
            review: anaesthetist/pharmacist with nurse
                discontinue: ward nurse
                feedback: patient!

Although it is to be hoped that everyone will have a good understanding of available methods of pain relief, it is least confusing in most cases if detailed discussion is left to the anaesthetist. The patient's notes should be studied carefully before going to the bedside, and the most informative section is often the exchange of letters between general practitioners and consultants. It is worth checking information about contacts with other specialties in addition to those implicated in the present admission. Above all, previous anaesthetic and recovery records may give useful information about previous analgesic treatment and side-effects. Clear introduction is needed so that patients can take in the name and function of the person who is going to be caring for them. Conveying an impression of limitless time is greatly helped by sitting down, preferably alongside the patient, so that the preoperative preparation is felt to be a joint activity. Probably the most important judgement that has to be made, and made quickly, is just how much information the patient wants. The patient needs time and 'space' in which to respond. An information sheet, as jargon-free as possible, should be available, and can be left with most patients, although a few may prefer not to have information thrust on them. The information sheet we use is reproduced in the appendix to Chapter 5.

Patient-care in the postoperative period gradually changes emphasis from the initial concern over recovery of consciousness and control of the airway and respiration, towards the recovery from the surgical insult and restitution of normality. In this chapter we will concentrate on ensuring that PCA, from establishment in the recovery room until discontinuation when the patient no longer needs narcotic analgesia, is used safely and effectively.

The distinction between these topics and the management of side-effects (Chapter 12) and the integration of PCA into overall postoperative care (Chapter 13) is necessarily artificial, but may aid concentration.

Nowadays it is becoming much more common for the management of anaesthesia to include various techniques involving the use of local anaesthetic drugs. We consider the ways in which this will affect the use and management of PCA in Chapter 14, and will here keep to the simplified situation of patients whose operation is to be managed entirely under conventional general anaesthesia. At the end of the book we have prepared some 'Quick Guides' that should be helpful for reference; two are for commonly encountered situations (1: Ward nurse taking over care of patient on PCA; 2:

Anaesthetist requiring memory-refreshment (However, if you are in any doubt about the operating procedures required on any machine, it is obviously essential to consult more senior staff or someone with previous experience of using it.) The third 'Quick Guide' (emergency treatment of severe respiratory depression) will, we trust, never be required for patients on PCA.

SMOOTH TAKE-OFF

We have suggested earlier that it is beneficial if narcotic administration is commenced during the operation, so that, on regaining consciousness, the patient is not starting from a zero blood level of narcotic. This will enable the patient to be brought to a comfortable state more quickly and/or accurately, whether intravenous titration by the anaesthetist is used or the patient achieves it by repeated activation of the PCA system. There are other advantages apart from the humane one of avoiding a period of possibly intense distress. There is evidence that, even under apparently adequate general anaesthesia, considerable activation of the stress response takes place (Kay *et al.* 1985) and may hinder recovery; these effects can be mitigated to some extent by giving pain-relieving drugs as part of a balanced anaesthetic technique. In addition, it has been suggested that central nervous system plasticity allows modification of the pain-receiving pathways and the state of surrounding areas so that less stimulus is required to produce pain perception after the initial painful stimulus (Tverskoy *et al.* 1990). Reducing the sensitivity to painful stimuli by the administration of opiates when such stimuli occur or immediately before appears to lessen the need for postoperative pain-relieving drugs. This effect has been termed pre-emptive analgesia (McQuay 1992). By contrast, the administration of narcotics in the absence of painful stimuli tends to produce a higher incidence of side-effects such as nausea and dysphoria; we do not therefore favour the use of narcotic premedication, but prefer to give opiates around the time of induction of anaesthesia. For most patients it seems simplest to use the same drug intra- and postoperatively, though there may be reasons for preferring shorter-acting drugs in particular patients, and the differences need to be taken account of during the initial treatment period.

The chosen PCA system will normally have been prepared during the operation, and it is connected, immediately on transfer to the recovery room, by the anaesthetist. For reasons discussed elsewhere we prefer to use a dedicated cannula and to secure and label it immediately. Concurrently the nurse will usually have made the initial routine observations of pulse rate, blood-pressure, respiratory rate, and oxygen saturation, as well as continuing supplementary oxygen, checking dressings, drains, and catheters, and connecting any additional monitoring needed. The PCA regime is then checked.

Although patients will have been given a reasonable account of the likelihood of postoperative pain and, usually, some introduction to the idea of PCA at the preoperative visit, we rely heavily on the recovery room staff to enquire sympathetically into their state as they wake up. Some will be pain-free, and therefore can be reassured, and can have the control system positioned and its method of use reiterated. Some will admit to 'a bit if soreness'—these we encourage to activate the PCA immediately, and then take assessment from there. All those with significant pain will be best treated by intravenous titration, and this is normally done by the anaesthetist responsible for the patient, using a separate syringe of the same drug via the injection port of the cannula being used for normal IV fluids. The increments chosen are usually two to two-and-a-half times the bolus dose selected, and at least three minutes would normally elapse before reassessing the patient's analgesic state. When the patients notice significant relief (not necessarily total freedom from pain) they are put in charge of the PCA and encouraged to take over activating it on their own judgement. The degree to which the average patient requires encouragement and reassurance that pain relief is good and suffering is of no physical or moral value should not be underestimated.

INITIAL ASSESSMENT

Patients who require very large amounts of additional opiate to bring them to an analgesic or near-analgesic state will normally have an immediate revision of the prescription and reprogramming of the machine to increase the bolus dose to a level likely to be satisfactory.

Because this is easy to do with electronic pumps we favour their use, and tend to start with small bolus doses to reduce side-effects in susceptible patients. If the fixed-volume Baxter device is being used one has to aim nearer the average effective bolus to avoid the likelihood of the patient's being unable to get sufficient analgesia with a reasonable dosing rate.

Clearly, if the anaesthetist is not going to be able to perform an initial titration because of other duties, or the response of the patient during the operation indicated that high doses were very likely to be needed, it is more sensible to choose a higher bolus dose at the first program setting. Several other factors can be taken into account in selecting a high bolus dose. These include the nature of the surgery—upper abdominal surgery is notoriously more painful on average than lower; youth and male sex, which both tend to make patients have high requirements and to be less likely to suffer nausea; and previous bad experience of postoperative pain or consumption of substantial quantities of analgesics over a long period (frequent in those with arthritic conditions). Above all, patients who are judged to be extremely anxious despite all efforts to decrease anxiety by giving full information are very likely to be high consumers of analgesic. On the other hand, a history of previous severe emetic complications makes it advisable to start with a relatively small bolus dose. Any patient with a history of postoperative nausea or vomiting (even minor) will probably benefit from an intravenous dose of metoclopramide either at the start of PCA or at the very first hint of nausea.

PHYSIOLOGICAL OBSERVATIONS ('VITAL SIGNS')

(a) In Recovery

In the recovery room the level of supervision, the routine frequency of observations, and the general concern for respiratory sufficiency are such that institution of PCA requires no additional observations. Recovery nurses are well versed in correcting minor degrees of obstruction and drawing the attention of the anaesthetist to irregular rate or depth. Pulse oximetry should now be used on all patients during at least the initial period in recovery. Monitoring of oxygen saturation by pulse oximetry allows good assessment of the need for supplementary oxygen and whether it can be discontinued before return to the ward. From the point of view of the effects of opiates, the judgement of when a patient is fit to return to the ordinary ward is made much easier by the use of PCA. Routine instructions for patients having IM opiates require a minimum period of 30 minutes' observation, whereas expiry of the lockout period is all that is needed before a PCA patient who is otherwise satisfactory can be transferred with confidence.

(b) On return to the normal ward

Although respiratory rate is routinely monitored, and has frequently been used as the principal indicator of respiratory adequacy (Notcutt and Morgan 1990; Wheatley *et al.* 1991), investigation has repeatedly shown that the rate and adequacy correlate very poorly—hypoxaemic patients can have normal or raised rates, and slow breathers may be doing perfectly well. This is admitted even by those who use rate as their chief indicator, and in a major report detailing the introduction of PCA into a DGH it seems that where slow rate was the only abnormality, action was never required for patients not receiving a background infusion (Notcutt and Morgan 1990). Enormous efforts were nevertheless put into making nurses undertake a taxing frequency of rate-counting. We see no point in seeking observations whose results we are almost certainly going to ignore, and prefer to encourage nurses to watch for respiratory obstruction, even minor degrees of which are worth correcting, and irregularity of respiration, which can indicate impaired respiratory control. This can be combined with the high level of general observation that we wish to encourage. At least for the first few hours after return, all postoperative patients should be in full view of the nursing station: a quick glance every few minutes is vitally complementary to formal recording of observations at specified intervals. Although it appears that PCA with modern equipment and careful protocols is at least as safe as conventional therapy, any system that connects a patient to a source of intravenous opiate has to allow for the possibility of accidents. We therefore do not allow any PCA patient to be in a side-room, and recommend two-hourly pulse-rate recording as the absolute minimum to supplement the standard four-hourly 'TPR and BP', which nurses are accustomed to modify using their clinical judgement. Some patients will need more observations (range and frequency), and these should be decided on clinical grounds. Instructions for observations which the clinician regards as mandatory as opposed to discretionary should be written down and signed.

RECORDING PAIN LEVELS

No formal assessment is made of pain level in the recovery room, since every PCA patient should be brought to a comfortable state; but we recognize that this is a counsel of perfection, and will not always be achieved, especially in those in whom residual drowsiness is apparent. Expediency often demands that their discharge cannot be indefinitely postponed when their general condition is satisfactory. The ability to keep a higher proportion of patients within a high-dependency area would greatly improve care in this type of patient. On return to the ward formal monitoring of pain levels should commence. This is desirable in all postoperative patients, and we have introduced a pilot scheme modifying the standard ward 'TPR' chart so that the area previously assigned to 'bowels, urine, and vomit' (!) allows recording of pain score on a 0 to 10 scale (see appendix to this chapter). The nurse shows the patient a large-scale, annotated pain 'thermometer' (Fig. 11.1) and the patient points to the level that accords with her or his present state; the numerical equivalent is then plotted on the chart. No assessment is made if the patient is asleep, and the chart is marked with the letter S. The assessment adds very little time to that required for the standard physiological observations, and rapidly becomes an acceptable routine. We believe it will improve patient-care whatever analgesic therapy is prescribed, and can form the basis for effective audit. Other workers have described satisfactory systems for pain-assessment by patients and nurses (Notcutt and Morgan 1990; Wheatley *et al.* 1991), and the addition of a factor that can distinguish between pain at rest and pain on movement appears particularly attractive.

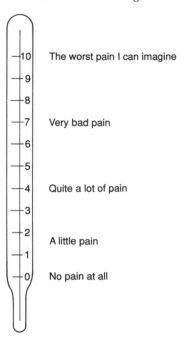

Fig. 11.1. A pain 'thermometer'.

OTHER NURSING PROBLEMS

Nursing staff at this time have to check that the patient and any visitors understand the PCA system and are clear about which is the nurse-call system. The handset should preferably be kept very close to the patient. If the patient's clothing needs changing, the pump does not need to be switched off. If necessary it can be disconnected, and this should always be done at the cannula. During manipulation, the cannula and the PCA line or Y-connector should both be protected by sterile caps or plugs (sometimes called blind hubs), which are cheap and readily available. A similar procedure can be followed if the patient needs to go to the X-ray department, if it is judged that analgesia will last well enough. The Baxter unit is especially suitable for very mobile patients—at least one patient of ours has been able to manage a shower!

REVIEWING THE PCA REGIME

All patients on PCA should be reassessed a few hours after their return to the ward. Ideally, this should probably take place three to four hours after discharge from Recovery, when surgical pain is likely still to be maximal and the residual effects of anaesthetic drugs have waned. There are several possible ways of organizing supervision, and some of these (and the reasons for adopting our own) will be discussed later in this chapter. For simplicity we will describe our present system, which seems to be an effective compromise. As near 6.30 in the evening as possible, the duty pharmacist finds out from Recovery the names and wards of all patients currently on PCA. Each ward is visited, and patients are reviewed with the senior nurse on duty. The prescription is checked against the equipment settings, the patients' most recent pain scores are noted, and they are asked how they are getting on with the PCA system. The intravenous site and the configuration of the connections are carefully checked, and an estimate is made of the rate of consumption by comparing the amount left in the syringe with the time since connection. This is also checked against the pump display of the amount consumed. A prediction of the time that the reservoir is likely to empty is then calculated (see Chapter 9). Any queries are dealt with, and specific enquiry is made about nausea and antiemetic administration, and about the possibility of the bolus dose's being too high (dizziness or nausea immediately after a request), or too low (inadequate analgesia or need for very frequent demands). It takes about fifteen minutes to assess each patient; but the total time taken for the round obviously depends on how many wards have to be visited and on the availability of appropriate nursing staff. At the end of the round, the pharmacist is able to ring either the duty or the consultant anaesthetist and make recommendations for each patient: on adjusting the bolus dose, on the effectiveness of antiemetics, and on the need to replenish the drug reservoir to avoid its running out during the night. Although individual drug consumption is relatively constant, a degree of diurnal variation has been found (Burns *et al.* 1989; Graves *et al.* 1983), with peaks in consumption around 9 a.m. and 8 p.m. Allowing for this, and for various other reasons, it is sensible to calculate the amount of drug needed to see the patient through until about 10 a.m. the next morning.

The anaesthetists can then plan to visit the ward either as soon as possible (where pain or nausea is a problem) or at a convenient time during the evening. The functions of the evening round are summarized in the box. The calculation of the likelihood of needing to recharge the drug reservoir has been dealt with in Chapter. 9.

Box 25. Check-list for the evening round

Check: patient: ? pain
                          ? nausea
                          ? using equipment OK

        : equipment: IV site
                       Connections/configuration
                       total used / consumption rate
                       'syringe empty' prediction

       : prescription: corresponds to equipment setting
                       antiemetics available/given
                       ?changes needed

any other problems.

This set-up works very well for patients operated on in the late morning or during the afternoon, but is clearly less than ideal for those returning from Recovery relatively early in the day or for emergencies operated on during the night. We are currently unable to extend to a regular morning review, although this is probably desirable.

ANTICIPATORY DOSING

Our ward nurses have been quick to perceive the great benefit of encouraging early mobility, and to maximize this by advising patients to administer a dose of analgesic in anticipation of getting out of bed or physiotherapy. The principle is well-established with IM analgesia, but the accuracy of timing and the absence of excessive effects that are possible with PCA are greatly appreciated. Removal of drains is another event that is viewed by all with greater equanimity when the patient is having PCA.

CHANGES IN PATTERN OF CONSUMPTION OR EFFECTIVENESS

Patients should be encouraged to discuss the effectiveness or otherwise of their treatment regime, so that changes can be appreciated and responded to at all times, although it is hoped that the routine round will allow adequate tailoring of programs to meet the majority of individual needs.

(a) Analgesia appears less effective

Sudden reduction in the effectiveness of analgesia can be detected either by increased demand rate or by the patient's pain level increasing or both. The two main possibilities are some form of system failure, or a change in the patient's condition leading to increased pain stimulus. A systematic check for the latter will include general observation of the patient's colour, respiration, and circulatory state, and of the operative site to eliminate surgical disasters, such as anastomotic breakdown or intestinal obstruction, the colicky pains of which are relatively unresponsive to analgesics. If the patient's clinical state appears unchanged the possibilities include cannula problems (tissueing or blockage), infusion line or connection blockage or misconnection, exhaustion of the drug reservoir, and inadvertent switching off of the machine. If blockage at any point is suspected it is best to disconnect the equipment from the patient before attempting to correct the fault, since pent-up doses may be released (this can happen even with well-designed equipment and appropriate alarms).

(b) Analgesia more effective or sedation excessive

As recovery progresses there is a natural diminution in the need for analgesics, and the patient may be transferred to oral therapy. Sudden increase in drug effect may indicate equipment malfunction—though this is extremely rare, and should become more so as improving pump design continues to eliminate sources of trouble. A more likely possibility is the onset of respiratory or circulatory problems that increase the sensitivity to opiates. Nevertheless, PCA is inherently relatively safe in situations such as hypovolaemia resulting from haemorrhage, although a bolus dose that is larger than optimal for a given patient may be sufficient to lead to depression if the blood volume is acutely reduced. In practice few problems have been experienced in distinguishing changes in clinical circumstances, despite the undoubted accuracy of Notcutt's perceptive statement (Notcutt and Morgan 1990) 'We found a natural tendency amongst staff to blame the new technique of PCA for a wide variety of routine postoperative complications.' Fortunately, this early suspicion is usually followed by enthusiasm, and the opposite problem of believing the technique to be a panacea for all ills is fairly easy to deal with!

DISCONTINUING THERAPY

The decision to transfer to less potent analgesics is usually made naturally and easily by the patient, with nursing-staff help if needed. Shortage of pumps usually means that some patients have to be deprived of PCA whilst they are still benefiting; this is a resource matter that is discussed in the relevant chapter. Premature discontinuation is less likely when a dedicated cannula is used, since there is otherwise a tendency to equate the end of need for IV fluids with the end of need for analgesia.

When the equipment is disconnected it is most important that the chart is completed, recording the date and time of termination, and the total dose of drug taken by the patient from the current reservoir, and thus the total consumed during treatment—this may also be read off the display of an electronic pump. The volume of solution remaining should be noted on the patient's chart. Finally the equipment should be promptly returned, complete with all accessories, to the Recovery Room. Here, the pump can be unlocked and the remaining solution discarded. The date of return and the volume of solution is recorded in the PCA diary

FEEDBACK FROM PATIENTS

Useful audit of the effectiveness and acceptability of PCA can be undertaken by a variety of means. We have principally used periodic questionnaires for this purpose, as well as to assess the usefulness and acceptability of our information sheets. Leaving plenty of space for additional comments often brings to light pockets of staff misunderstanding (for example 'I was told to use it as little as possible'), and highlights some things that on occasion distress patients more than pain (for example, noise on the ward at night). Interviews may not necessarily be more informative, since at interview patients may conform more to what they perceive as the desired responses; they are certainly more time-consuming.

OTHER WAYS OF ORGANIZING THE SUPERVISION OF PCA

We acknowledge that what we have described is probably the minimum supervision that should be accorded to patients on PCA.

Were more resources available the following possibilities would be explored, either separately or in combination.

(a) Rounds by consultant anaesthetists

Regular morning and evening rounds by consultants, with sessional allocation of time for acute pain control, could deal with all necessary changes in therapy on the spot, and ensure that staff training and documentation continued correctly. Alternatively, rounds could be undertaken by the on-call consultant.

(b) Other grades of anaesthetist

In many hospitals, anaesthetists on standby for emergencies (particularly obstetrics) have sufficient unoccupied time to make it reasonably certain that they could undertake supervisory rounds within a reasonable period of time.

(c) Specialist nurses

Employment of acute-pain-control nurses with suitable training and experience could allow supervisory rounds as well as involvement in training other staff and optimizing care with methods other than PCA.

(d) Recovery-room nurses

The familiarity of recovery-room nurses with the equipment and the fact that they introduce the majority of patients to the technique suggest that they could visit patients on the wards at appropriate times and perform the necessary checks. This requires an increased level of staffing in Recovery to allow for absences while on such visits.

Our use of pharmacists has been prompted by their interest and enthusiasm in clinical care in general and PCA in particular, and by their necessary presence on duty with relatively light duties at the time most appropriate for an evening round.

APPENDIX: A MODIFICATION OF THE STANDARD WARD 'TPR' CHART TO ALLOW RECORDING OF A PAIN SCORE ON A 0 TO 10 SCALE

Name		Bed No.
Ward	Unit No:	

MONTH															
DAY															

F	C	AM	PM	AM	PM	AM	PM	AM	PM	AM	PM	AM	PM	AM	PM
05·8°–41°		2 6 10	2 6 10	2 6 10	2 6 10	2 6 10	2 6 10	2 6 10	2 6 10	2 6 10	2 6 10	2 6 10	2 6 10	2 6 10	2 6 10

104°–40°

102·2°–39°

100·4° 38°

98·6°–37°

96·8°–36°

95°–35°

PULSE

170
160
150
140
130
120
110
100
90
80
70
60
50

RESPIRATION

40
30
25
20
15

PAIN

8
6
4
2

12 *Minimizing side-effects*

Using opiate drugs to relieve pain inevitably brings their side-effects into consideration. By individualizing the dose for each patient in relation to his or her pain experience over a short period of time there can be no doubt that PCA will produce the best balance between effective analgesia and those side-effects that are merely unpleasant for the patient, since she or he can choose reasonably precisely what that balance shall be. There are some indications that dangerous side-effects are also minimized; but we must not let our intuitive belief in this likelihood run ahead of the proof that only further research backed by wider clinical experience can bring.

The side-effects attributed to opiates include nausea, with or without vomiting; respiratory depression; depression of gut motility; sedation; and other central effects, such as euphoria, hallucinations, and convulsions. The increase in understanding of opiate receptors and the development of newer drugs suggests that it may eventually be possible to produce a non-nauseating opiate, since it has certainly proved possible to produce some that are much worse than the old ones! However, the mixed agonist/antagonists have a ceiling for respiratory depression that appears to be parallelled by a ceiling for analgesic effect, and whether respiratory-depressant potential can ever be eliminated is still academic: for the present and foreseeable future we must use what is available.

Box 26. Principal side-effects of opiates

- Nausea and vomiting
- Respiratory depression
- Reduced gut motility/smooth-muscle spasm
- Sedation
- CNS stimulant effects

NAUSEA AND VOMITING

These are central effects, aggravated by the reduction in gastric emptying. There seems little to choose between the three drugs best suited to PCA, although diamorphine may have some advantage (Dundee *et al.* 1966). Editors may groan at the request for more research into dealing with nausea and vomiting; however, there is little doubt that patients regard it as at least as important as pain. Whilst PCA allows us to be confident in reassuring our patients with regard to pain control, until we can treat emetic sequelae effectively this will remain its single greatest drawback. Since the effect is dose-related, the advisability of keeping the PCA bolus dose to the smallest that produces an adequate degree and time of analgesia should not need reiterating. The many causes of nausea seem to be additive, and therefore attention to all such matters will reduce the opiate effect. General measures that will reduce the tendency to nausea and vomiting include avoiding prolonged starvation, hypoxia, or hypovolaemia.

Box 27. Factors affecting postoperative nausea and vomiting

- Premedication
- Anaesthetic management
- Postoperative nursing care
- Antiemetics

Preoperative factors

Many people will feel nauseated simply as a result of missing a meal; over 50 per cent of female subjects are likely to experience nausea if fasted for 7 hours (Palazzo and Strunin 1984), and the rigid adherence to the traditional preoperative 'nil by mouth after midnight' will produce adverse starting conditions. It is manifestly impossible for all patients scheduled for the morning list to have their operations at 8.30; but individualized regimes will be resisted as long as a cavalier approach to altering list order is allowed to continue. A conscientious anaesthetist who has tried hard to minimize restriction of preoperative oral intake by prediction of induction time and appropriate ward instruction will feel aggrieved and embarrassed when greeted at 8.30 a.m. in the anaesthetic room by the patient scheduled to be last on the list. Sharpening up theatre management may yet improve the patient's lot in addition to efficiency (Bevan 1989). Few would argue that the elective patient requires more than four hours' restriction of oral intake prior to induction (or opiate premedication), and studies have shown that prolonged fasting does not guarantee an empty stomach (Hester and Heath 1977). Since the point of the restriction is to lessen the risk of aspiration of gastric acid it is time to consider combining the proven effective regimes for reducing the volume and acidity of gastric contents (Popat *et al.* 1991) with more liberal preoperative regimes for which there is already evidence of low risk (Miller *et al.* 1983). Small trials have shown satisfactory results (Maltby *et al.* 1988); but altering everyday practice depends on more than science.

Premedication

Opiate premedication may induce nausea in sensitive subjects, and any desirable effects on induction of anaesthesia can be achieved by intravenous administration at the time. The most likely effect is to increase the total dose received by the patient without any increase in analgesia. In addition, staff time for checking and administration is much greater than for oral premedication, and many patients greatly dislike injections.

Diazepam and other tranquillizers used for premedication are associated with a lower incidence of postoperative nausea and vomiting than opiate premedication (Haslett and Dundee 1968), and this is a further reason for deprecating the continuing use of preoperative opiate injections. Increasingly, H2 receptor blockers are used to ensure safe levels of acidity in gastric contents. Although it is not clear whether this also reduces postoperative nausea and vomiting, it certainly reduces the unpleasant taste if you do vomit!

Anaesthetic management

Propofol appears to have less emetic potential than other intravenous anaesthetic induction agents. Some patients seem to be susceptible to nitrous oxide (possibly because of its effects on the middle ear (Thomsen *et al.* 1965)), and may benefit greatly from its avoidance—even if they require more intraoperative opiate for analgesia! A degree of dehydration is probably inevitable in some patients, and the young fit person having a minor but painful operation may be helped by IV fluids, even though operative blood loss is negligible and prompt resumption of oral intake is confidently predicted (Cook *et al.* 1990).

Immediate postoperative factors

One other important detail—both noise and movement greatly intensify nausea, and should be reduced as far as possible (Kamath *et al.* 1990). Many recovery rooms permit excessive noise and bustle to accompany necessary activity, and the numerous visitors on postoperative wards should not be allowed to increase noise levels. A further benefit that might result from high-dependency units would be the reduction in the need to move patients at a stage which can be critical for the degree of nausea engendered—a long bumpy trolley ride can be the last straw.

Treatment

Nausea is undoubtedly undertreated. Most anaesthetists prescribe antiemetics 'prn': patients frequently receive nothing until they actually vomit, if then. We have stressed the importance both of prescribing them and checking that they have been given appropriately whenever the PCA regime is reviewed. The practicability of adding nausea scoring to the standard observations should be considered. As with pain, reluctance to treat symptoms regarded as not dangerous in themselves must be tackled.

Antiemetics that are commonly used act mainly on the chemoreceptor trigger centre in the brain, although metoclopramide also acts by speeding gastric emptying. Hospital formularies have reduced the range of these drugs available, and in addition to metoclopramide our standard drug is prochlorperazine. We are yet to be convinced that preoperative administration of antiemetics has much effect on postoperative events. The most effective way to use metoclopramide, in our experience, is to give a 10 mg IV bolus at the first hint of nausea; we explain preoperatively that 'Some people still have a tendency to feel sick; if you feel at all nauseated you must tell us immediately, because that gives us the best chance of treating it successfully—it simply isn't worth hoping it will go away.'

Data sheet recommendations for dose and dose-interval of antiemetics are, in general, very cautious, because of the undeniable risk of extremely unpleasant extrapyramidal side-effects. We feel however, that the distress caused by nausea and vomiting must be weighed against this. We have felt justified in being more liberal, bearing in mind the very large doses of metoclopramide recommended for prevention of the emetic side-effects of cytotoxic therapy, since the loading dose for this regime (2–4 mg/kg over 15–30 min) equates to 10 mg/min intravenously for a 75 kg person. Our standard prescription for IM metoclopramide (10 mg 6-hourly, prn) remains close to the recommended dose; but we no longer hesitate to supplement this with additional IV boluses.

If this is ineffective we change to prochlorperazine, 12.5 mg IM 6-hourly prn, although we are not particularly impressed with the results, and are interested in the suggestion that prochlorperazine is associated with a very high incidence of nightmares in the postoperative period. The addition of an antiemetic to the opiate solution will ensure concurrent administration of a dose with each bolus. A preliminary study has shown some promise (Williams et al. 1993); however, the potential for overdosage of antiemetic in patients with high opiate requirements is a disadvantage.

Acupressure and acupuncture are undoubtedly effective (Ghaly et al. 1987), though rather brief in their action, and deserve more extensive trial. Acupressure should be applied at the P6 point—3 fingersbreadths above the proximal palmar skin crease, beside the palmaris longus tendon. Patients can be taught self-application preoperatively if they have had bad experiences previously. It is then important that they are not prevented from using the technique by the siting of IV cannulae.

The use of ginger root taken orally at the time of premedication has shown promising evidence of effectiveness (Bone et al. 1990); the preparation has no recorded side-effects (unlike all other antiemetic drugs), and clearly deserves further study to see whether its effects will summate with drug therapy.

In the near future, we would like to assess much more aggressive antiemetic regimes, adopting perhaps the high-dose metoclopramide therapy used by oncologists for patients on cytotoxic treatment. The newly-introduced antiserotonin agent, ondansetron, is undergoing intensive evaluation as a perioperative antiemetic, and we await conclusions with interest. The more impressed we become by the effectiveness of PCA in terms of pain control, the more distressed we are by the suffering of those whose nausea and vomiting are not successfully treated.

RESPIRATORY DEPRESSION

Opiates tend to reduce the rate and depth of breathing when given to normal subjects. Patients in pain are protected to some extent from these effects by the stimulus of their pain, which, untreated, can lead to hyperventilation, as is exemplified by the response to normal labour. However, where pain is itself produced by deep breathing, as after abdominal or thoracic operations, suppression leads to an increase in pulmonary infection rates. The respiratory effects of opiates in the postoperative period are further complicated by the possibility of residual sedative and respiratory-depressant effects of anaesthetic agents and incomplete return of full muscle power after muscle-relaxants, although all these are much less of a problem with modern anaesthetic techniques than they used to be. Hypoxaemia is also increased by ventilation—perfusion abnormalities associated with anaesthesia and surgery. The ability to monitor oxygen saturation continuously in the peripheral circulation has made it possible to focus on episodic respiratory problems (Rosenberg *et al.* 1989), and we have become more aware of the contribution of obstruction (Hanning 1989). Overt obstructive sleep apnoea is relatively rare except in obese subjects; but even minor degrees of snoring, when superimposed on disordered sensitivity of the central control of respiration, become important in the postoperative period (Reeder *et al.* 1991*a*). Recent work has emphasized that, following major surgery in an at-risk population, hypoxaemia is commonly worst on the second and third postoperative nights; that tachycardia and hypertension are often associated; and that myocardial ischaemia and infarction are probably causally related (Reeder *et al.* 1991*b*). For a given level of effective opiate analgesia, PCA is accompanied by less risk of respiratory depression than other methods of administration

(Wheatley *et al.* 1990), presumably because it minimizes fluctuations in blood level and tailors the blood level to the pain stimulus accurately. We have outlined in Chapter 11 the reasons for regarding respiratory rate as an unsatisfactory routine detector of respiratory depression and our preference for general observation, supplemented wherever possible by pulse oximetry. Patients who have pre or intraoperative indication of respiratory problems may still be best treated by PCA; but the level of supervision must be appropriate, and may require the facilities and staff levels of an HDU or ITU.

Combining other methods of pain relief, particularly those involving local anaesthetic agents, can lead to overt respiratory depression if the extra analgesia is superimposed on an already adequate blood level of opiate: by 'unbalancing' the equation between pain stimulus and respiratory depression the depressant action of the opiate may become dominant (McQuay 1988). One possible way for this to happen is if it is decided to reinstate an epidural block that was used at operation, but was allowed to wear off in favour of PCA.

The incidence of respiratory problems requiring intervention in patients satisfactorily established on PCA and returned to the ward is very low unless background infusions are added, and this is our main reason for advising strongly against their use. Other possible causes of depression from relative overdosage include demand-switch activation by relatives or nurses, and malfunction or misconnection of the equipment (Wheatley *et al.* 1991; Grover and Heath 1992; Notcutt *et al.* 1992). Use of a dedicated cannula will reduce misconnection problems, although 'hi-jacking' for other purposes is difficult to eliminate. Careful attention to initial setting up, and a regular check of configuration to ensure that the intravenous infusion is protected by a one-way valve if a Y-connector is used, must be adhered to.

A patient who is awake, breathing easily and regularly, and with a good colour is unlikely to be depressed: any departure from this easily recognizable, desirable picture needs to prompt an appropriate reaction from the observer. It is surprisingly difficult to determine a logical sequence of responses so that the patient is safe but not needlessly disturbed, and the staff can feel confident that they are neither crying 'wolf' nor running risks. Well-managed wards and recovery rooms certainly do not produce enough instances of the various grades of respiratory problem to allow all staff to be trained apprentice-style, acting under supervision and being judged safe to cope with all eventualities before having to take first-line responsibility. This has to be understood and faced up to by trainers and trainees alike, and is a good reason for regarding a period spent in direct contact with anaesthetic practice as desirable for all nursing and medical staff. Discussion, simulation, and 'what would you do if' scene-setting has to supplement routine experience.

The lowest level of concern should be generated by a slow respiratory rate: when this is detected, the most important first response should be to check conscious state and colour. Assuming a good colour, if the patient appears awake, then asking him or her to take a deep breath checks responsiveness, the presence of a clear airway, and muscle power and co-ordination; if asleep, observation of the character of respiration (whether regular and unobstructed) should allow the observer to be reassured without necessarily rousing the patient. Where a minor degree of obstruction can be seen but patients rouse easily and are otherwise satisfactory, they should be encouraged and assisted into a comfortable position in which the airway remains clear without assistance.

Irregular breathing in a sleeping patient will occur during periods of rapid-eye-movement (REM) sleep; however, this sleep pattern tends to be suppressed during the immediate postoperative period, and therefore at this time it is more likely to indicate some degree of disordered respiratory control, and should lead to careful appraisal of the patient's condition.

Apnoeic episodes (Catling *et al.* 1980) are clearly dangerous. It seems that mild or moderate hypoxaemia can intensify the effects of opiates on the respiratory centre, since the administration of supplementary oxygen can lead to improvement in ventilatory control without alteration in the level of analgesia, which is however the inevitable accompaniment of drug treatment. Any suspicion of cyanosis requires immediate action: encouragement to deeper breathing, rousing if necessary, and administration (or repositioning) of supplementary oxygen should be automatic, and, unless resolution is prompt, summoning help and checking saturation with a pulse oximeter.

IMPLICATIONS FOR WARD EQUIPMENT

We foresee increasing interest in improving patient care by extending monitoring in the postoperative period. At present, a reasonable minimum requirement for a surgical ward should be access to ECG and pulse oximetry. This can be achieved by dedicated ward equipment or by borrowing from a central stock. We would advocate a combination: each ward should have its own ECG and oximeter, and should be able to obtain further items as soon as any patient requires continuous monitoring. The ease of application of the oximeter makes it an ideal method of rapid checking of what is probably the most vital physiological function. Although the current generation of pulse oximeters are prone to false alarms when used on unanaesthetized patients, because of motion artefacts, technological development should overcome this problem, and thus allow a much greater acceptance of pulse oximetry on ordinary wards. Confidence in safety is essential to confidence in analgesia.

GUT MOTILITY

Opiates reduce gut motility, causing constipation and gastric stasis. These undesirable effects have dangerous aspects: regurgitation and aspiration of stomach contents may be rendered more likely, and bowel anastomoses may be endangered (Aitkenhead and Robinson 1989). If the evidence for the difference in potential for this latter problem between morphine and pethidine is confirmed this will be a stimulus for examining the mechanism by which the difference is mediated. It seems likely that the reduced incidence of anastomotic dehiscence in patients receiving pethidine is related to its spasmolytic effects, and the addition of spasmolytic drugs to a morphine-based analgesic regime may be required for at-risk patients. As was previously discussed in Chapter 3, there are other good reasons for not recommending pethidine for PCA. Further evidence for the possibility of serious consequences arising from muscle spasm is provided by a case report in which the use of morphine via PCA appears to have caused pancreatitis as a result of spasm of the sphincter of Oddi (Mills and Goddard 1991).

Attention to symptomatic relief of nausea is likely to minimize gastric stasis, since metoclopramide restores motility. Good nursing care will maintain an alertness to the distress of constipation and ensure optimal management.

SLEEP DISTURBANCE AND SEDATION

The importance of sleep to the patient's well-being and speed of recovery is one of the most important and most neglected aspects of postoperative management and research. Patients after major surgery will frequently volunteer their feelings that recovery did not really start until they had their first 'proper' sleep, often after a miserable 24–48 hours of intermittent dozing, wakefulness, and drugged stupor. Opiates tend to destroy normal sleep patterns, abolishing REM sleep. Patients who are deprived of REM sleep for periods of about 48 hours appear to have a compensatory increase, often associated with ventilatory disturbance, central apnoeic attacks, and episodic hypoxia. It has been suggested that the increased incidence of myocardial infarction in the third postoperative day may be related to this phenomenon. Clinically, patients receiving PCA appear to achieve better sleep patterns, and this may be related to the optimization of dosage and reduction in anxiety; more specifically, the steady reduction in blood level of opiate once the patient falls asleep (often cited as a theoretical disadvantage of PCA) may decrease the opiate-mediated interference with sleep pattern. Further research into this area is needed; but it seems likely that this may prove to be one of the mechanisms by which the general recovery of the patient is aided by PCA.

Sedation is an acknowledged side-effect of most opiates, which is usually welcomed by patients. Before the introduction of PCA, attempts at improving postoperative pain relief in Lewisham Hospital centred on intravenous infusions. These often provided excellent analgesia in the early postoperative period for young patients, but required a good deal of fiddling with to get the right sort of rate. Older people were so often unsatisfactorily managed in this way that the technique was abandoned on normal wards. It seemed quite common for such patients to be oversedated but still complaining of pain. PCA has not presented this problem, and this seems to indicate that small fluctuations in blood level are necessary to good results. These observations are probably a variant of the reasons for the unsatisfactory results of supplementing PCA with background infusions.

The newer synthetic drugs such as fentanyl are very much less sedative, and could be considered for patients who very much dislike feeling at all muzzy.

EFFECTS DUE TO CNS STIMULATION

Hallucinations, euphoria, dysphoria, and even convulsions have all been described in certain circumstances with most of the opiate drugs. These effects are more common after the mixed agonist/antagonist drugs such as pentazocine. We have not seen any evidence of such reactions with our PCA regimes. Clearly, such effects might manifest themselves in susceptible patients, perhaps as a result of drug reactions. After excluding other causes, simple sedation with small amounts of diazepam could be used.

13 Patient-controlled analgesia as part of overall postoperative care

In this chapter we draw together some of the ways in which PCA can contribute to the last two of the aims of perioperative care that were identified in Chapter 2:

- minimizing the effects of physical and emotional trauma;
- returning the patient as rapidly and as far as possible to independent full function.

The physical impact of surgical trauma includes the activation of physiological compensation mechanisms for many systems whose normality has been disrupted in some way: blood and fluid loss (direct and by evaporation and sequestration) is added to fluid deprivation during the preoperative period, and stresses both cardiovascular and renal systems; loss of temperature-control intensifies heat-loss, and metabolic compensation in turn imposes demands on the respiratory and circulatory systems; tissue damage evokes intense neural activity, both directly and as a consequence of the release of active chemicals; and the resultant pain and muscle spasm can start a vicious circle of metabolic demand. In simple evolutionary terms, the reaction to trauma may be thought of as primarily directed towards salvaging only those individuals likely to be able to resume contribution to the survival of the species. The young person reacts to moderate blood loss and tissue damage—perhaps a fall causing a long bone fracture—by intense vasoconstriction, which minimizes blood loss, and by muscle spasm, thus reducing movement and allowing healing to occur. If trauma is more extensive the intensification of all the reactive mechanisms is actually harmful, and contributes to the demise of the subject—perfectly efficient and reasonable in evolutionary terms. Human development has led to a wider view of the value of individuals, and the care team therefore has to devote a good deal of time, effort, and ingenuity to reducing the harmful components of physiological responses to the trauma that we deem it reasonable to inflict on individuals for their long-term benefit!

It is only recently that there has been any widespread general acceptance of the idea that treating pain is really important to the recovery process. Many people have argued on humanitarian grounds, and some have identified psychological and emotional interactions; but the collective medical ethos has relegated the practicalities of pain relief to nursing staff, and accepted a responsibility for the prescription of drugs mainly as a medicolegal necessity. Nursing staff have been left in an awkward role as a result; the stress laid upon the dangers of opiates has been complicated by the small degree of responsibility given to them. The introduction of more effective techniques for pain relief has prompted a more honest acknowledgement of the degree of suffering, and studies that we have referred to elsewhere throughout this book are starting to document both the benefits of better postoperative pain control and the mechanisms by which they may be brought about. It becomes increasingly plausible to suggest that neither doctors nor nurses should have the prime authority in managing pain: their role can be thought of as an enabling one, allowing provision of safe and effective regimes in which the patient is the prime mover.

Patient-controlled analgesia can restore patient autonomy, thus reducing anxiety; and this in turn will reduce the overall requirement for pain relief. The individualization of dosing requirements allows the best chance of reducing both side-effects and the metabolic burden on drug inactivation and excretion mechanisms. It has allowed demonstration of the diurnal variation in drug requirements, which has been shown to peak around 8–9 in the morning and to be at its lowest in the early hours of the morning (Burns *et al.* 1989); no other method of administration can so easily or accurately follow the individual's needs. This accuracy, together with the sense of control, are particularly important in breaking the vicious circle that can develop as anxiety and pain interact. It has been noted that, whilst preoperative anxiety is very important as a determinant of pain experience, anxiety actually peaks in the immediate postoperative period. Fears about the significance and success of the procedure are compounded by worries about complications. It is at this time that staff have plenty of practical tasks to attend to: observations, dressings, intravenous infusions, and antibiotic administration, for example. It is very easy to forget that patients are just as anxious for information and reassurance. They should be encouraged to articulate all their fears, so that the appropriate explanations and support can be given. Many patients have little understanding of how their bodies work, and can suffer great distress from the most bizarre imaginary complications—a process that can be fuelled by media obsessions with the more dramatic side of health care, and by insensitive relatives and friends.

Anaesthetists and recovery room staff have little difficulty in accepting the reality of the wide differences in pain experience and analgesic requirements after similar surgery. Back on the postoperative ward there may be a strong tendency to view susceptibility to pain as somehow indicative of 'lack of moral strength'. There is no doubt that it is a very natural reaction to blame the patient for the failure of a therapeutic maneouvre, and traditional analgesic regimes have reinforced this pattern strongly. PCA, because of its convenience and effectiveness and because differences in consumption are not obvious, can help to correct this outlook, although it will probably never be completely eliminated. One point deserves emphasis: the length of time that patients experience pain after particular procedures is also variable, and pain relief should be continued for as long as is needed, with suitable variation in the type of analgesic. Also, some surgery that produces very little physiological disturbance may be very painful; and these are both further reasons for dissociating PCA from intravenous fluid administration. In the future we may even see adaptation of PCA to allow patients to use it at home, thus extending the range of procedures acceptable for day-care.

PCA must be seen, however, as only one of a number of ways of dealing with pain; and therefore the concept of the Acute Pain Team has been introduced (Notcutt and Morgan 1990; Wheatley *et al*. 1991). This undoubtedly has great potential for the improvement of management so that each patient will have a considered regimen, with regular supervision.

Although PCA eliminates the need for intramuscular injections of analgesics, its use often requires antiemetic injections, and these can cause distress. Kluger and Owen (1990) found that the absence of injections rated sixth in the categories of advantages for PCA perceived by patients. About 10 per cent of adults are needle-phobic, and will avoid making any complaint that will result in an intramuscular injection. Not only are an even higher proportion of children and adolescents similarly affected, but the problem is compounded by nursing staff's reluctance to even suggest injections to them. For both these groups we strongly recommend the insertion of an intramuscular cannula into the thigh during anaesthesia (Teillol-Foo 1991). This is secured and labelled, and the recovery and prescription charts are duly annotated: 'give all IMI via cannula in left thigh, aspirate before injecting'. Patients for whom this is relevant are identified preoperatively, and have the system explained to them; they derive great reassurance from knowing that 'the nurse will put the needle into the plastic, not into you'. It is necessary to use a cannula without a one-way valved injection port, so that aspiration can be used to detect inadvertent intravascular placement: we favour 'Y-cans', whose injection 'eyeball' is designed to protect the nurse from the risk of stabbing herself with the needle. The currently available models are rather short for obese patients, but it is likely that this problem will soon be overcome. Where the only drugs likely to be required by injection are satisfactorily absorbed from subcutaneous tissues, the anterior abdominal wall may prove a more convenient and comfortable site.

CHANGES RESULTING FROM THE INTRODUCTION OF PCA

As the number of anaesthetists interested in PCA has increased and enthusiasm for its use has spread amongst nursing staff, attention to the general condition of patients on postoperative wards has been increased: replacing the long-standing regime of intramuscular injections prn. prompted very reasonable concern to ensure that the new 'improved' treatment did not represent a significant danger. The fact that this has coincided with the availability of much-improved pulse oximeters and the familiarity of anaesthetists and recovery staff with this continuous monitoring has made it easier for research workers to study oxygenation in the postoperative period.

Reduction in arterial oxygen tension postoperatively was well docu-mented in the 1960s (e.g. Nunn and Payne 1962), and the associations with age, smoking, respiratory disease, and site of surgery were noted. Nunn and his colleagues drew attention to the ventilation—perfu-sion abnormalities which, combined with reduced cardiac output, intensified the effects of other factors. Postoperative oxygen supplementation was frequently recommended, but rarely persisted with beyond a few hours unless the patient was cared for in an ITU. The advent of oximeters now means that hypoxaemia is less easy to ignore.

SUPPLEMENTARY OXYGEN

Recent evidence (Wheatley *et al*. 1992; Madej et al. 1992) suggests that PCA produces fewer, less severe episodes of hypoxaemia, and a more stable pattern of oxygen saturation than epidural or intramuscular opiates given to comparable analgesic levels. These interesting studies have not confirmed the suggestion (Wheatley *et al*. 1990) that preoperative oximetry might be a useful predictor of patients susceptible to an unstable pattern of oxygen saturation, and therefore particularly likely to benefit from the closer supervision possible within a high-dependency unit. There is little doubt that more patients should have supplementary oxygen for longer than is current practice—many studies (for example Marshall *et al*. 1972) have indicated that postoperative hypoxaemia is common, and not necessarily accompained by hypercarbia (or vice versa). Increasing use of pulse oximetry has drawn attention to the frequency with which intermittent hypoxaemia can occur (Catley *et al*. 1985), and the possibility that episodes may be related to myocardial problems (Reeder *et al*. 1991*b*). The practical problem lies in devising acceptable techniques for prolonged administration of supplementary oxygen under ordinary ward conditions: one video surveillance study (Nolan *et al*. 1992) of the first postoperative night in 20 patients showed that the oxygen mask remained on and correctly positioned throughout in only one patient. We recommend that each ward is supplied with a pulse oximeter, so that nurses may at the very least check saturations whenever they suspect a respiratory problem. It may be possible to add a pulse oximeter reading to the standard set of observations—it takes less time and affords at least as valuable information as the blood-pressure. Nasal cannulae or spectacles may prove to be more satisfactory and acceptable methods for oxygen therapy. It seems likely that most patients over 55 undergoing major surgery would benefit from supplementary oxygen, particularly at night, and that it should be continued at least for the first three nights. This has little specifically to do with PCA, but is an area of postoperative care that will benefit from increased attention (see Hanning 1992 for an excellent review of this subject).

POSTOPERATIVE CHEST INFECTIONS

One of the reasons that patients may, on average, leave hospital sooner if they have received PCA is a reduction in postoperative pulmonary problems. The mechanisms may be earlier and better mobilization, so that fewer infections start, or better co-operation with physiotherapy, so that they clear more quickly. The role of physiotherapists is very important, and they should be included in the education programme when PCA is introduced: they rapidly recognize the benefits, and often initiate referrals to the Acute Pain Team.

RESUMPTION OF NUTRITION

Nutrition in postoperative patients is not given the attention it deserves. Whilst there are many reasons for this, PCA may play a minor role in improving matters by reducing the time spent by nurses checking and giving injections and by optimizing the dosage of opiates so that the return of normal gut function is encouraged.

14 Integration of PCA with other methods of postoperative pain relief

The recent focus on postoperative pain relief and its inadequacies has raised awareness of the wide variety of techniques and drugs that can be brought to bear on the problem. Some of these techniques seek alternatives to the traditional drugs, some are different ways of using opiates and local anaesthetic agents, and others seek to modify troublesome side-effects.

Evolution of clinical practice is dependent on the activities of enthusiasts who hope to convert, or at least influence, conservatives. Conservatism may be deemed a polite term for lack of vision, imagination, motivation, or energy; it is nevertheless, on occasion, a necessary curb on uncritical promotion of novelty. The combination of a naïve clinician with a thrusting commercial organization can produce results that may be seductive, but may prove not to be in the best interests of the majority of patients, or may be disastrous for a few. Pressure for research publications where funds are difficult to raise increases the possibilities for distortion. We are enthusiasts for PCA, and freely admit that our clinical experience of other specialized techniques is very limited. In spite of this, we feel there is value in drawing together a brief review of other methods, and indicating those areas where combinations offer a hopeful prospect.

Box 28 illustrates the matrix of agents and possible routes of application that we have heard of—it is unlikely to be comprehensive.

Given this amazing variety, the aspects that we will consider include effectiveness, safety, and applicability. Closely interrelated with these are the issues of resources: both for equipment and specialist (medical, nursing, or pharmacy) time. Given unlimited time and resources one might produce safe, perfect pain relief for virtually all patients; to carry this to a ridiculous extreme (for purely illustrative purposes) one would need perfect psychological/personality matching for patient, therapist, and treatment regime, since even the most skilful attention will not produce satisfaction if it involves having to suffer the frequent presence of someone you find

Box 28. Analgesic treatments

d = described. ++ = reasonably useful postoperatively

Agent:	opiate	NSAID	LA	electricity	α-adrenergic agonists	other
Route:						
oral	++	++				
inhaled	d					
rectal	d	++				
IM	++	++				
IV	++	d	d		d	
infiltration			++			
nerve block	d		++			
regional	++		++		d	
transdermal	d	d	d			
TENS				++		
Acupuncture				++		++
Hypnosis						++

unpleasant or irritating! The serious point underlying this is that, in addition to the importance of the patient's personality, which has been discussed at length in Chapter 4, the effect of personality interactions can influence results of drug treatments, particularly in the field of information-giving and routine pain assessment. This is probably a major reason for the failure to replicate in everyday practice the results obtained by the enthusiast.

OPIATES BY OTHER ROUTES

Oral

The ease and familiarity of giving drugs by mouth make it the obvious choice for treating mild pain, and many attempts have been made to extend this, especially by the introduction of long-acting (sustained-release) preparations of opiates such as morphine. Success in treating chronic pain has stimulated attempts to use these preparations for postoperative pain; however, the time-characteristics of the pain and the analgesic method are fundamentally mismatched—using the oral route to build up an adequate blood level is slow, and interference with gut function results in great variation. Low blood levels when pain is at its height are likely to be followed by excessive levels later. The best that might be hoped for is the production of a background level that will synergize with other methods in the early postoperative period. The place of these preparations (for example morphine continus and Aspav—a combination of aspirin and papaveretum) in pain relief after day-case procedures has not been fully explored, and it seems likely that they have considerable potential for mitigating a serious problem.

Intramuscular

A great deal has already been said about the comparison between nurse-administered on-demand intramuscular injections and PCA. There is certainly nothing to be said for any combination of the two systems. One study (Welchew 1983) compared a regular intra-muscular regime (4-hourly morphine) with on-demand fentanyl, and found no difference in pain relief; but this is likely to relate to choice of fentanyl for PCA. Given the variability of individual needs, rigid regimes are inherently unlikely to be either safe or effective in acute postoperative pain. This is in marked contrast to their use in chronic pain, where appropriate dosage can be carefully titrated, and is unlikely to change at all rapidly; the full benefits of well-timed regular regimes in preventing the recurrence of pain can be realized in this setting.

Spinal and epidural

The direct application of solutions of opioids to the spinal cord and nerve roots, via either the epidural or spinal route, results in excellent analgesia, which is usually prolonged. Some studies (for example Estok *et al.* 1987) have shown no difference in analgesic consumption when on-demand analgesia via the epidural route was compared with intravenous PCA; however, Welchew and Breen (1991) appeared to show a marked reduction in consumption via the epidural route. Both these studies used fentanyl, whose characteristics are probably better suited to the epidural route. The latter study provoked trenchant comments (Kluger and Owen

1991; Ali *et al*. 1991) and equally brisk responses (Welchew 1991 *a*, *b*), demonstrating some of the problems in interpretation of studies. A factor not raised as yet is the major distraction/extra attention factor that must have been generated by the study's assessment techniques. Although with both the spinal and epidural route there may be a contribution from the effects of systemic absorption and subsequent central action on higher centres, it is clear that the majority of the effects of epidurally administered opiates arise locally. Some side-effects are minimized—euphoria or sedation; some reduced—nausea and hypotension; and some intensified—itching. Respiratory depression has proved to be an extremely variable and unpredictable problem, with reports of late onset of severe depression (Davies *et al*. 1981), which have prompted consideration of the possibility of cephalad spread of opiate within the cerebrospinal fluid; but another possibility is that waning of painful stimulus with time uncovers respiratory-depressant effects—it is too often forgotten that an equation exists between the central reception of painful stimuli and the actions of opiates, and that levels of analgesia and respiratory depression are the resultants. Summation with opiates administered by other routes can be a problem. Most anaesthetists would feel that the level of supervision required for patients receiving repeated doses of spinal or epidural opiates necessitates admission to a High-Dependency or Intensive Care Unit. The system also takes a substantial period of time to set up, and the anaesthetist reponsible, far from being able to slot this into a relatively inactive part of the operative period, has to give the patient his or her undivided attention (thus suspending the activity of the rest of the surgical team), and may even require to be supported by a second anaesthetist. These factors mean that the technique is favoured for patients with high-risk combined surgical and medical conditions, for whom it represents the optimal solution.

Combined opiate-local anaesthetic regional techniques

There is growing evidence that combining low doses of opiates and local anaesthetic agents by infusion can minimize the disadvantages of both, and provide high-quality, safe analgesia for high-risk patients within the setting of a general surgical ward (Wheatley *et al.* 1991). It is of interest that in the first year of operation of an Acute Pain Service utilizing both PCA and EIA (extradural infusion analgesia) with this combined technique, Wheatley *et al.* reported even better pain relief with EIA (average VAS pain scores for 150 EIA patients—2.2; for 510 PCA patients—3.5), but a slightly lower level of satisfaction (91 per cent vs 96 per cent satisfied); both these results were statistically significant, $p < 0.05$. Dissatisfaction with EIA was ascribed to lack of control, reduced mobility, urinary retention, and some technical failures. Problems were also noted with hypotension from relative hypovolaemia.

Intravenous infusions

Intravenous infusions of opiates are commonly used for seriously ill patients as part of intensive care, particularly for those requiring artificial ventilation, when respiratory depression is almost an advantage. They can provide more satisfactory postoperative pain relief than intramuscular injections, for the obvious reason that fluctuations in blood levels from intermittent and variable absorption are eliminated. Careful monitoring and safeguards on equipment design are clearly mandatory. We see two areas where it does not compete with PCA: the lack of a sense of control and the inherent inflexibility of the regime, which does not allow the patient to anticipate painful events and does not automatically reduce intake during sleep, when needs are reduced, perhaps by attenuation of anxiety. Patient-controlled infusions hold out the promise of 'smoothing' requirements; but, particularly in the elderly, it seems extraordinarily difficult to achieve good analgesia without excessive sedation; this fact combined with the lack of success with background infusions as part of a PCA regime leads us to postulate that *some* fluctuation (within quite small limits) has a valuable effect, possibly owing to a 'switching' effect. Hill and colleagues (1991) have shown better results with a pharmacokinetically based patient-controlled morphine infusion regime than with conventional PCA in a group of patients suffering from oral mucositis pain during bone-marrow transplantation. This type of pain may differ significantly from postoperative pain; but there was also a substantial difference in the initial stages of therapy, which ensured that the patients on the infusion regime rapidly achieved a target blood level (via a bolus dose and pharmacokinetically-tailored rapid infusion), whereas the conventional PCA regime patient could only build up slowly from normal bolus doses (1–2 mg morphine, 10 min lockout), which required staff to adjust the limits only if *they* judged them to be insufficient. This difference is reflected in the mean hourly consumption rates, which were only about one-quarter those of the infusion regime on the first treatment day, and never reached half during the study period: the PCA patients would have had to press the button every 15 min (on a 1 mg bolus) throughout the 24-hour period to achieve an equivalent consumption on the first day. The 30 per cent reduction in pain intensity reported could well be accounted for by this much greater uptake of morphine. Although the investigators thought that they had ensured access to as much morphine as the PCA patients felt they required, we feel that they may have overlooked the effect that having to articulate an increased requirement to staff has on patients. Without patient-monitoring at a level at least of that in an HDU, variability in the patients' condition, particularly their haemodynamic status, renders IV infusions potentially more dangerous than other systemic administration methods.

Transdermal and inhalation

Trials of these somewhat exotic routes seem to have resulted from extending the findings of relative efficacy and convenience for drugs such as glyceryl trinitrate and salbutamol, for which more common routes pose particular problems. Despite 'encouraging results' (Rowbotham *et al.* 1989*b*; Higgins *et al.* 1991) they seem most unlikely to achieve an important place in postoperative pain relief.

NON-STEROIDAL ANTI-INFLAMMATORY DRUGS

It is certain that the potential of this class of drugs has not yet been fully explored; a relative newcomer, ketorolac, has shown promise in several studies (Burns *et al.* 1991; McQuay *et al.* 1986; Honig and Van Ochten 1986), and both naproxen and diclofenac are becoming relatively widely used. What is also not fully understood is the range or significance of the possible side-effects which can arise as a result of their mode of action, which is basically interference with the prostaglandin system.

The study by Burns *et al.* is a model of the use of PCA as an investigative tool to determine the effectiveness of ancillary drugs. They showed that a continuous intramuscular infusion of ketorolac reduced morphine uptake from a PCA device by approximately half during the first 24 hours following upper abdominal surgery; however, no patient was sufficiently analgesic not to use the PCA at all (minimum uptake 24 mg), and this confirms the trend in all studies of these agents—that they may provide valuable adjuncts, and thus reduce undesirable side-effects, but are not a complete alternative to opiates.

Suppository preparations are extremely useful, as they are rapidly absorbed and act for a prolonged period; the traditional reluctance to use the rectal route is easily overcome by seeking the assistance of the scrub nurse, who can insert the suppository before removing his or her gloves when the patient is turned on his or her side immediately before recovery from anaesthesia. Since the intramuscular route is particularly painful, we feel it need not be used.

LOCAL ANAESTHETICS

Simple infiltration of skin incisions is increasingly practised by surgeons, and helps to reduce the intensity of pain immediately after awakening from general anaesthesia. It might be thought that it would interfere with the introduction of PCA in the recovery room by removing the requirement for analgesia. This has not been our clinical experience: the technique seems only to mitigate one element of pain after the types of surgery for which we recommend PCA, and does not normally lead to the patient's having any difficulty using PCA even without prior introduction.

The type of surgery performed under nerve-block techniques will not usually merit PCA where there is a limited number of pumps available. Regional blockade has been discussed under opiate therapy, since combinations of opiates and local anaesthetics are becoming more popular. The local anaesthetic contribution may add further complications, since migration of epidural cannulae to the subarachnoid space may result in the catastrophic advent of high spinal block. We repeat the warning proffered by McQuay (1988), who drew attention to the possibility of opiate-induced respiratory depression's occurring if total pain relief was produced by any form of neural blockade in a patient already receiving morphine. This could happen if PCA were to be rejected by a patient, either because of inefficacy or side-effects such as nausea and vomiting, and regional blockade instituted.

NON-DRUG TREATMENTS

Acupuncture and hypnosis may be useful methods for particular patients; they require training and enthusiasm on the part of the practitioner, and the normal UK surgical patient is unlikely to view them with much favour. We have no experience of them, but do not reject them as ancillary methods for the future. Hypnosis appears to require very time-consuming preoperative preparation.

   The value of the Acute Pain Team will doubtless increase as a greater diversity of methods enters their repertoire.

15   Our research with PCA

Our views on the psychological aspects of pain control and the practical management of patients using PCA are closely bound up with the studies that we ourselves have carried out. This research is fully reported in Thomas (1991) (a Ph.D. thesis), but is not yet published elsewhere, apart from one abstract (Thomas *et al.* 1990). We therefore concentrate in this chapter on these studies, and do not aim to review general research carried out with PCA, much of which is referred to in other parts of the book.

IMPETUS FOR THE RESEARCH

The impetus for the research came from a general desire to gain an understanding of the origin of pain, since this could have important consequences for the experience of pain and hence the design of a system to relieve it. For example, two people may have identical surgery, but the experience of pain may be totally different, depending on the reason for surgery or the background history of the injury (Barrier 1985) and the personality of the patient. The success of PCA may also be influenced by these factors.

Another aspect which prompted our research is the limited availability of PCA, owing to its cost. The future of PCA lies in balancing the clinical success with the economics involved, and it seemed to us that the most satisfactory way forward would be to put the psychology of the patient into the equation. Maynard (1987) defines the economics of health care as 'the science of deciding how to allocate scarce resources'. The achievement of economic efficiency requires the minimization of cost and the maximization of outcomes. With regard to PCA, it is difficult at the present time to reduce initial cost significantly, but it is possible to maximize its use and potential benefits. Methods must be developed that will reduce inefficiency.

Essential to the efficient use of PCA is an understanding of the categories of patients for whom it will be most effective. A consequence of the limited availability of PCA systems is that choices have to be made, and it is important to consider the criteria that will be used to choose which patients will benefit most from their use. At present, however, understanding of the factors which could be used as bases for decisions is extremely limited and unclear. Frequently, anaesthetists use the extent of trauma as a guide, although there is no clear evidence that this is the most effective strategy. Moreover it ignores the numerous psychological factors which empirical research has shown to influence acute pain. As was explained in Chapter 4, these include state and trait anxiety (Johnston 1986), neuroticism (Taenzer *et al.* 1986), and coping style (Wilson and Bennett 1984; Miller 1980), as well as situational factors.

The research now to be discussed therefore evaluated these patient variables in order to determine which patients derive the greatest benefit from PCA.

EXPERIMENTAL DESIGN

A total of 164 female and male patients undergoing elective cholecystectomy, hysterectomy, laparotomy, and hip replacement were investigated. Preoperatively, all patients were assessed in terms of state and trait anxiety, neuroticism, and coping style by means of standard, validated questionnaires (respectively Spielberger State/Trait Anxiety Inventory, Eysenck Personality Questionnaire, and Miller). Postoperative pain assessments (using Short form McGill Pain Questionnaire including VAS) were made at 6, 18, and 24 hours after surgery. Patients were allocated to receive papaveretum for analgesia either by PCA or by IMI on demand from nursing staff. A subset of 40 female patients received a very-low-dose background infusion from the PCA pump in addition to either PCA or IMI prn, to investigate the possible placebo effect of the equipment's presence. The total quantities of drug administered and the length of hospital stay were recorded. Estimates of time expended on pain relief and assessment of the views of staff and patients were also undertaken. Statistical analyses included T tests, analysis of variance, and multiple regression.

SUMMARY OF FINDINGS AND IMPLICATIONS

Psychological variables

Anxiety (both state and trait) and neuroticism were all found to influence pain for both PCA and IMI. Moreover, the relationship was essentially similar for both regimes: high levels of all factors being associated with high levels of pain. The highest correlations were with state anxiety. However, there was a difference between the regimes in terms of the relationship between coping style and postoperative pain experience, with a positive relationship being shown for IMI and a negative relationship for PCA. This difference suggests that patients with low-monitoring coping style scores tend to experience more pain using PCA than those with high-monitoring scores; whilst with IMI, the low-monitors did better than those with higher scores. Since high-monitoring style reflects a desire for control, this finding suggests that such patients are more likely to achieve maximal benefit because they prefer to be in control, whereas low monitors may not achieve such efficient pain relief when using PCA because they do not like to exercise the control that it gives them. This finding has implications for determining those who might derive the greatest benefit from PCA.

Pain scores and drug consumption

However, it must be emphasized that the overall findings of the studies confirmed the substantial and significant superiority of PCA over IMI in all groups, despite the greater consumption of papaveretum by the latter method (PCA vs IMI, mean total pain scores: 20.22 vs 36.48, mean papaveretum mg 57.08 vs 83.59).

Most important factors

When patients were divided according to their anxiety scores, it was found that the relief achieved with PCA was greater for the high-anxiety group than for the group with low levels of anxiety.

These results suggest that the patients who benefit maximally from PCA are those with high levels of preoperative anxiety and those with high-monitoring coping styles. Conversely, the patients who will benefit relatively less are those with low anxiety levels and those with low-monitoring coping styles.

Length of stay

In addition to better pain control, PCA was also associated with a mean reduction in length of stay of 2 days. Thus the beneficial effects of PCA potentially have considerable economic implications for the NHS. The current costs of maintaining a patient on a surgical ward are estimated to be over £200 per day, and if this reduction in hospitalization becomes a consistent finding among PCA patients there could be a considerable financial saving for individual hospitals to set against the costs of the PCA system, which are estimated at about £20 per patient treatment episode. This matter is considered in more detail in Chapter 10. As well as financial savings, there could be an important effect on surgical waiting-lists.

Placebo effect from background infusion

There was no evidence for a placebo effect related to the presence of the sophisticated PCA equipment. Despite the very low dosage chosen (*c*.0.5 mg/hr), the background infusion resulted in higher total drug consumption, with no improvement in pain scores.

Time-saving element

PCA can save time while patients are in hospital, because the amount of nursing time required to provide postoperative analgesia is considerable. This study compared the time expended for both methods of analgesia.

Twelve trained nurses were asked to assess how long it took to administer intramuscular injections and the length of time it took to carry out safety checks on patients using PCA systems over a four-week period. The results showed that IMI takes an average of 11.5 minutes to perform, compared to 4.5 minutes for the PCA checks, and this represents a saving of 42 minutes per patient per day.

Views of patients and staff concerning PCA

Questionnaires were completed by patients, nurses, and anaesthetists. These revealed a high level of enthusiasm for PCA amongst all respondents; some details are presented below.

Patients

Of the seventy patients who completed the evaluation questionnaire, none reported any difficulties in using the device. Indeed, one of the things they liked about PCA was its ease and simplicity of use. The aspect which most appealed to them was that they did not have to bother the nurses for their pain relief. This finding allays the concern that has been expressed (Dodson 1985) that patients using PCA may become worried because they are not getting enough attention from nursing staff. The word 'bother' was used by many patients, and suggests that they consider the provision of pain relief an unnecessary nuisance for the staff, a finding also highlighted by Seers (1987). Overall, patients felt very good about being in control of their pain relief, and there were no fears about overdose.

Nurses and anaesthetists

Fifteen nurses and five anaesthetists completed the evaluation questionnaire. All staff thought that PCA was much better than IM injections in controlling pain, and they considered putting the patient in control to be a positive move. All but one of the nurses particularly liked PCA because it released them from the time-consuming task of checking controlled drugs for IMI. However the nursing staff felt that they required more education about the principles of PCA.

On the negative side, the nursing staff disliked the bulkiness of the PCA machines, which made it difficult to change patients' nightclothes. The anaesthetic staff, on the other hand, were more concerned with the fact that there were insufficient PCA systems, for reasons of cost.

FUTURE RESEARCH TO BE UNDERTAKEN

A predictive criterion

A long-range objective lies in developing an easy-to-administer questionnaire which could be used in the allocation of PCA facilities. As a preliminary stage, multiple regression analyses have been carried out on the actual responses to individual questions in the assessments for state and trait anxiety, neuroticism, and coping style, in order to find those questions most predictive of pain experience. Nine questions have been identified, and it is expected that some of these will form the core of the questionnaire. Additional objective information, such as patients' age, gender, and cultural background would be included. After validation of the items in this instrument, it is anticipated that a numerical scoring system might be derived to provide a rating of expected postoperative pain. This in turn could be used as a criterion for allocating patients to available PCA systems. It may also prove possible to identify a group of patients for whom an IMI regime can provide acceptable analgesia.

16 The future: clinical developments and research

Research works best, or at least more easily, when it is directed at a few well-defined questions. Clinical research tends to be somewhat messy—a balance struck between restricting the problem to make the conclusions statistically valid and widening it sufficiently to make the conclusions clinically useful. The many published studies carried out on PCA to which we have referred freely throughout this book range around this balance. Overall, it is clear that PCA has been found effective and safe; however, some of the results are conflicting, and the discussion of them is bound to reflect the authors' attitudes and preconceptions as well as their findings. It is not our brief to conduct a comprehensive review nor yet a critique; but it may be of value to examine some of the ways in which discrepancies can arise, and to explore factors that can influence results and their interpretation. Many of these factors are common to all research on patient treatment, and will therefore be treated briefly; others are pertinent to studies of analgesia and PCA in particular. This discussion is aimed towards both those who carry out studies and those who read and are influenced by the reports.

AVOIDANCE OF BIAS

The well-recognized sources of bias in patient-selection for studies are boring in their familiarity: age, weight, sex, type and length of surgery, premedication, anaesthetic technique—it can be viewed almost as a game to see if anyone (ourselves included) has missed an obvious one. Less commonly attended to are ethnic origins and social and educational factors: small studies relying on questionnaires are heavily dependent on literacy skills, and even we were surprised by an anecdote illustrating the fact that some people regard 'mild' pain as worse than 'moderate'. Refusal to take part in or dropping out during a study can also introduce bias, particularly in psychological characteristics, and the reader must be in a position to assess this possibility.

TEMPORAL FACTORS

Time of day, time of year, and actual date can all be important. It is fairly obvious that outcomes in groups of patients are most easily compared if they are studied over the same time-period and on the same wards, because the ethos of care is continuously evolving, and in different ways amongst different staff groups; similarly, diurnal variations can affect results. Anaesthetic techniques evolve, and the analgesic component can vary markedly from one anaesthetist to another. Theatre lists are often constructed to a fixed pattern, with major cases placed early, and most anaesthetists try to do cases requiring epidurals first; it may not be practical to change this, but at least the investigator and reader should be aware of it. The crucial thing is to record everything that is done very accurately, so that where the ideal cannot be achieved the possible effects of any departure can be faced and assessed. At any time after the completion of a study, other work may raise questions that can be answered if comprehensive records have been kept.

PLACEBO EFFECTS

The effects of special equipment and extra attention must be borne in mind; they are very difficult to eliminate without producing circumstances that bear little relation to normal practice. The essence of both PCA and IMI prn. regimes is a decision to initiate medication, either by the nurse or the patient. Since the treatments have completely different time-courses of action there is no scope for the patient to receive both treatments, with one being inactive and neither nurse nor patient knowing which. It is therefore not possible ethically to construct a strict, double-blind trial of PCA against an IMI prn. regime, although it can be compared to a regime of regular, fixed-dose intramuscular injections. The latter is difficult to make both safe and reasonably effective, because of the variation in requirements—which is no doubt why it is not a common clinical regime for postoperative pain.

INFORMATION

It must be possible to assess the information offered to patients about the pain-relief schemes which they may receive, since this can have major effects on their perception of treatment and thus on anxiety levels. A healthy scepticism has to be maintained in this area, because of the extraordinary sensitivity of interpersonal relationships: striking the wrong note can prejudice the most carefully planned informative interview, and psychological research techniques require substantial special training.

SPECIFICATION OF PCA REGIME

When it comes to the 'mechanics' of a PCA regime there can be many important variations. Achieving a satisfactory level of analgesia at the start of treatment must happen quickly: any regime which allows a patient to wake with unmodified pain and relies on the normal dosing scheme to reach analgesia will get results so inferior to those which can be achieved in normal clinical practice that interpretation is prejudiced.

For patients to have the benefits of a true sense of control, the lockout period must not be too long, either as a result of poor programming or apparatus deadspace effects. It is noticeable that more recent reports are specifying 'dedicated cannula, bolus dose x, lockout y, no background infusion' rather than merely 'patients received morphine on demand via PCA'; this is an admirable trend. Clearly, the inclusion of a background infusion has such important effects (on total drug consumption and respiratory depression) that it must be noted and considered. When results are quoted in terms of drug consumption (especially for drugs with which one is not very familiar and when expressed in mg/kg body weight) it is a useful exercise to convert this into terms which give a clear clinical picture: try converting the drug into morphine equivalents, the dose into that which a 70 kg patient would receive, judging the bolus dose for appropriateness in the target population, and then calculating how often the patients at the extremes of the range had to press the button to reach their consumption. This allows you to assess whether some patients were getting very big doses infrequently or having to demand doses immediately the lockout expired, thus turning them into desperate 'clock-watchers' or frenetic button-pressers. Some unexpected results become easier to understand when trouble is taken to obtain a clear picture of events.

FUTURE DEVELOPMENTS

We feel confident that the provision of patient-controlled analgesia for healthy adults undergoing major surgery will become widespread (we hope the norm) in the immediate future. There are areas of practice where PCA may be the optimum analgesic regime for a greater or lesser proportion of the relevant surgical population. The definition of these areas has to be by research and careful reporting of clinical experience: we would restate the fact that results obtainable under the special conditions of clinical research are not always translatable into routine practice.

(a) Paediatric practice

Many children have to undergo painful surgery. Where the pain is relatively short-lived, after tonsillectomy for instance, the complexity of PCA is not indicated, although application of the principle of exact individual titration (via the intravenous route) to a comfortable state immediately postoperatively will do much to relieve distress and improve the perception of hospital care by children and their parents. Surgery followed by a more prolonged painful period merits PCA wherever sufficient expertise can be built up to manage the somewhat more complex situation that results from the necessary involvement of parents. Parents need to function primarily as interpreters, but sometimes as agents, for the child. Staff have to judge how well the parents can cope with these roles, and how much help and encouragement they need in understanding all aspects of the postoperative scene and in acting appropriately. Research is needed to assess the best strategies in terms of safe, effective analgesia and in terms of the cost-effective use of equipment and special skills. Units specializing in trauma and orthopaedics, burns, and correction of congenital or acquired abnormalities that require repeated surgery are clearly best placed to develop and audit progress; they need to secure funding to ensure that the maximum knowledge derived from their experience can be diffused out to other more generalized services.

There are two particular questions that we would like to see studied. Firstly, the appropriate drugs, dosages, and regimes for the very young. Secondly, the interaction of opiate analgesia and the autonomic system in children. The latter area interests us because of the recognized difference in autonomic (particularly vagal) balance in children, which has led many anaesthetists to retain modest atropine premedication for children long after abandoning it for adults. The opiates vary in their autonomic effects: for instance, morphine is generally a vagal stimulant, whereas pethidine is vagolytic. It is pertinent that, amongst the remarkably few reports of adverse effects of uncomplicated PCA, two have been in children, one (Mills and Goddard 1991) where morphine via PCA seems to have precipitated spasm of the sphincter of Oddi, and another (Mowbray and Gaukroger 1990) which draws attention to the difficulty experienced in controlling colicky abdominal pain. It may be that the higher vagal tone in children makes them more susceptible to the effects of morphine on smooth muscle, and there may be a need to undertake specific treatment to mitigate this.

(b) Psychological aspects

In the preceding chapter we have described work that we have carried out and the extension that we hope to undertake on identifying the most appropriate patients for PCA. There is still interesting work to be done on tailoring both analgesia regime and the style and content of information to patients' psychological profiles. An increasingly consumer-orientated health service and professional interest in audit may give impetus to studies in this area, and even do some of the work under other headings.

The measurement of pain has advanced enormously in recent years, helped by the widespread acknowledgement that the patient is the best person to assess its severity. A number of pain-assessment tools have been developed which are aimed at enhancing people's verbal expression of their suffering so that they can convey their subjective experiences. The simplest techniques are the unidimensional verbal rating scales and visual analogue scales (Green 1990). Verbal rating scales consist of a sequence of words corresponding to escalating pain. A simple verbal rating scale asks the patient to rate the pain as none, mild, moderate, or severe. Scores obtained in this way are difficult to use for statistical comparisons because the change in pain intensity represented by the difference between, for example, 'none' and 'mild' may not be the same as that between 'moderate' and 'severe', and it is not therefore possible to produce a meaningful average. Visual analogue scales (VAS) consist of a straight line, usually 100 mm in length, with the ends representing the extreme limits of pain—'none' and 'unbearable' (Scott and Huskisson 1976). Such scores are assumed to be amenable to statistical tests for parametric data: i.e. the degree of change in pain-intensity represented by a particular distance (for example 5 mm) is assumed to be the same however far along the line it is placed, so that the difference between a mark at 24 mm and one at 29 mm is taken to represent the same degree of intensification of pain as the change between 43 mm and 48 mm. This allows simple averages to be calculated and compared. The pain 'thermometer' seems to be an easily understood presentation of the VAS (see Chapter 11). Numerical rating scales are a variant form, in which patients are asked to score pain intensity from 0 to 10 (as opposed to the freedom to place a mark at any point along the 10 cm line). They are regarded as easy to use (Seymour 1982), but are probably not as good as the VAS.

The use of these unidimensional scales (allowing the patient to express a variation in intensity only) do not reflect the complexity of pain experience, and Reading (1984) has argued that over repeated trials patients may use single scales to reflect different components of their pain according to the aspect that most concerns them at a particular moment. Methods have been developed which allow pain to be scaled in three dimensions: sensory-discriminative, motivation-affective, and cognitive-evaluative. The best known multidimensional method is the McGill Pain Questionnaire (MPQ, Melzack 1975). It has been extensively tested and used, but is far too time-consuming for use in the postoperative situation. A shortened form—the SF-MPQ—has therefore been developed (Melzack 1987), enabling rapid acquisition of data. It is easy to administer, and provides information on sensory and affective components as well as on the overall intensity of pain.

Ideally, the assessment of pain should also include time of onset and its impact on normal basic activities such as breathing and movement. Although it may appear more troublesome to record pain scores under two sets of conditions (at rest and on movement) it can actually make it easier for the patient to decide on the intensity that he or she feels represents his or her condition, and is therefore recommended both for research and clinical purposes.

Although pain-assessment is fundamental to research into pain, other psychological measures are certain to yield important findings contributing to a better understanding and management of postoperative pain. Further work is needed on clinically applicable methods of preoperative identification of factors, such as anxiety and coping style, that have been demonstrated to affect pain experience. Successful, practicable methods of modifying these factors both pre- and postoperatively need to be evaluated.

(c) Gastrointestinal effects

The effects of opiates on the gut are important in adults as well as children. Constipation is a well-acknowledged side-effect of morphine that can interfere markedly with postoperative recovery, although it is to some extent counteracted by mobilization, which is helped by good pain relief. This is an area which would benefit from the attentions of research nurses. A surgically important topic is to elucidate the effects of opiates after bowel surgery, both on resumption of motility and on the incidence of anastomotic problems. The excellent results of the epidural route may produce a fine balance in the choice of optimal technique: PCA is certainly cost-effective, but may have a disadvantage if it exposes the patient's intestine more directly to the effects of opiates. On the other hand there may be ways of reducing the effects, and the comparison of morphine and papaveretum may yield answers.

Nausea and vomiting still persist as the most disliked sequelae of PCA, and effective regimes (preferably not involving intramuscular injections) are urgently required. Whether the answers lie with acupuncture, ginger root, fixed- or variable-dose intravenous infusions of antiemetics (phenothiazine, butyrophenone, antidopaminergic, or antiserotonin) or the elimination of nitrous oxide remains to be seen—the group eliminating this problem would merit a Nobel prize.

(d) Alternative routes

Although we have confined our attention to the intravenous route, there is clearly scope for more extension of the principle of patient control. Studies of the epidural route to complement those already undertaken should address the topics of supervision, drug combinations, mobility, and urinary retention.

(e) Day surgery

Since postoperative pain is one of the factors limiting day surgery, investigations into the feasibility and safety of a 'take-away' service should be undertaken. This could be done by simulating home conditions initially on an ordinary ward and subsequently in a 'self-care' facility within the hospital site. The cost of a disposable PCA device compares very favourably with the cost of a hospital bed over 24 hours, and even an ultracautious approach to total drug dispensed and to patient-selection could still produce interesting results. The pressure to reduce length of hospital stay often results in patients who have undergone fairly extensive, but superficial, surgery being discharged at a time when pain is still severe; techniques developed for day surgery could clearly also alleviate much distress for other short-stay patients.

(f) Postoperative complications

There are firm indications that the use of PCA is associated with a reduced length of stay. There is a clear need to identify the associations with common postoperative complications such as thromboembolism and chest infection and the interaction with improved mobilization.

(g) Staff development

The promotion of patient-controlled analgesia is an opportunity for the involvement of several disciplines in further understanding of many important factors in postoperative care. Clinically important research can help the development of a multidisciplinary team approach which can benefit staff as well as patients. Current emphasis on audit will encourage this evolution.

QUICK GUIDE 1: CHECK-LIST FOR WARD NURSE TAKING OVER PATIENT ON PCA
(This assumes that general postoperative state is satisfactory.)

- Is the patient comfortable now?—Read the prescription, it should tell you how much of what drug she or he may take and how long she or he must wait before obtaining another dose.
- Is the patient nauseated?—Have antiemetics been prescribed and/or given?
- Has the patient activated the machine by herself or himself?
- One press or two required?
- If appropriate, is the pump plugged into the mains and indicating 'running' or 'ready'?
- Is there plenty left in the syringe/reservoir?
- Is it clear who you should call if:
  (a) the syringe needs refilling?
  (b) you are unhappy with the patient's condition?—for example, if analgesia or antiemesis is inadequate; if there is oversedation or respiratory depression (the house surgeon is responsible for matters related to the surgical condition).
  (c) the machine indicates a fault that you cannot correct? (Most pumps have an 'alarm' switch to press—this temporarily stops the noise and lets you think. The screen should tell you what the problem is; there may also be a reset button that you have to push when you have solved the problem—otherwise press 'stop' and then 'run' or 'start' again.)
- If the problem is occlusion (of the cannula) press 'stop', disconnect at the cannula, and flush with 2 ml 0.9 per cent saline—take care to check with a second appropriate person. Press lightly over the end of the cannula whilst removing the syringe and reconnecting the pump to ensure that the cannula does not refill with blood. Some pumps (for example, the Graseby 3300) require the syringe cover to be unlocked and the pump drive released and refitted before the pump will restart; therefore you will have to call someone with a key.

QUICK GUIDE 2: FOR ANAESTHETISTS REQUIRING MEMORY-REFRESHMENT

This assumes:

(1) that you are familiar with the principles of PCA;

(2) that you have read the Hospital or Departmental PCA Policy and/or Protocols carefully; and

(3) that you have received supervised instruction previously, and have the operating instructions for the device in front of you.

**IF NOT,
DO NOTHING WITHOUT APPROPRIATE
SUPERVISION AND HELP.**

Baxter infuser

You have to provide the motive power by distending the silastic reservoir. The lockout is 6 minutes, and cannot be varied. Decide the bolus you want to give and prepare a 60 ml syringe of drug whose concentration means that the bolus is contained in 0.5 ml for example (morphine 1 mg bolus, therefore 2 mg/ml, therefore 120 mg morphine in 60 ml). Follow the instructions for filling the reservoir: it cannot be done very quickly, because it takes quite a lot of pressure; similarly, priming the tubing and the control 'wristwatch' cannot be hurried, because the fluid is only released at 5 ml **per hour**. Make sure you do not have air in the syringe and that you follow the correct order of filling—the reservoir first; then allow its connecting tubing to fill; then attach the control module and allow it to fill till it drips; then remove the shipping insert to allow the dose reservoir to fill; depress once to expel any remaining air; and then replace the cap until ready to connect to the patient—it will be 6 minutes before he or she can take the first bolus. Stick the dose indicator on the side of the housing, lining it up carefully.

Electronic pumps

Check whether the pump runs on mains with battery back-up, or on batteries alone. If mains, plug in and switch on. Check syringe type and size, and fill with the chosen drug at a concentration that will make the bolus dose at least 0.5 ml; attach the line (and a one-way valve connector unless you are using a dedicated cannula) and prime manually. Write the prescription, and have an experienced nurse check your calculations and syringe preparation. Attach the label away from the markings. Follow the menu prompts or manufacturers' instructions to program. Do not use the purge facility or the loading dose. Do not use the background infusion or time drug limits (x mg total allowed in y hours) unless there are very special reasons. Pumps which require the latter to be programmed should have a default setting which is equivalent to the maximum allowed by your choice of bolus and lockout (for example: bolus 1 mg, lockout 6 min, one hour maximum = 10 mg). When the program is complete, load the syringe (take care that the graduations are visible), close the cover and lock, and check that the pump indicates that it is ready to run. If necessary, switch off at the mains, unplug, and take to the patient (this will not wipe the program: the pump will run on its internal battery during transfer).

Whichever device is used:

(1) Get the patient comfortable (or very nearly) with intravenous increments of your chosen drug from a separate syringe: use about twice your bolus dose (or more if they are clearly in agony), flush in well, and wait only 3–4 minutes between increments if they are in severe pain, or 4–5 minutes if you think you are nearly there.

(2) Give intravenous metoclopramide if the patient is at all nauseated.

(3) Connect the PCA line: **either** direct to a dedicated cannula, **or** to the sidearm of the valved connector, attach the IV infusion to the valved port of the connector and flush through, and then connect it directly on to the cannula to minimize deadspace.

(4) Hand over to the nurse and check that she or he is experienced in encouraging patients to use the handset appropriately.

QUICK GUIDE 3: Emergency treatment of severe respiratory depression due to opiate overdose

(This may be caused by malfunction of equipment, major programming or drug preparation errors, or activation of PCA by someone other than the patient.)

- The Patient will be unresponsive, with pinpoint pupils and respiration either absent or greatly reduced in rate and or depth.
- If this is not the picture, consider other causes of collapse.
- **If no pulse is palpable, commence cardiopulmonary resuscitation and call the cardiac arrest team.**
- Turn off and disconnect PCA. If cardiac output is adequate give oxygen, and assist respiration if necessary. Give **naloxone** 3 micrograms/kg IV (usual adult dose = 200 micrograms, this is **0.5 ml** of the 1 ml ampoule of Narcan, which contains 400 micrograms; the 2 ml ampoules contain 2 mg—2000 micrograms—and are intended for dilution—only 0.2 ml is therefore required for a bolus); repeat at 2-minute intervals until a satisfactory response is obtained.
- **An IV infusion** will usually be needed if massive overdose has occurred: dilute either a 2 ml ampoule or five 1 ml ampoules in 500 ml of normal saline (4 micrograms/ml) and titrate the dose to keep the patient satisfactory—usually this means with a respiratory rate > 10/min.

REFERENCES

Adams, A.P. and Pybus D.A. (1978). Delayed respiratory depression after use of fentanyl during anaesthesia. *British Medical Journal*, 1, 278–9.

Aiken, L.H. and Henrichs, T.F. (1971). Systematic relaxation as a nursing intervention technique with open heart surgery patients. *Nursing Research*, 20, 212–17.

Aitkenhead, A.R. and Robinson, S. (1989). Influence of morphine and pethidine on the incidence of anastomotic dehiscence after colonic surgery. *British Journal of Anaesthesia*, 63, 230–1P.

Ali, S., Digger, T.J., and Perks, D. (1991). On demand epidural fentanyl. *Anaesthesia*, 46, 984.

Anderson, E.A. (1987). Preoperative preparation for cardiac surgery facilitates recovery, reduces psychological distress and reduces the incidence of postoperative hypertension. *Journal of Consulting and Clinical Psychology*, 55, 513–20.

Andrew, J.M. (1970). Recovery from surgery, with and without preparatory instruction, for three coping styles. *Journal of Personality and Social Psychology*, 15, 264–71.

Angell, M. (1982). The quality of mercy. *New England Journal of Medicine*, 306, 98–9.

Annan, F.J., Ray, D., and Drummond, G.B. (1988). Comparison of rate of onset of respiratory depression after IV morphine or diamorphine. *British Journal of Anaesthesia*, 61, 112P–113.

Arntz, A. and Schmidt, A.J.M. (1989). Perceived control and the experience of pain. In Stress, personal control, and health (ed. A. Steptoe and A. Appels), pp. 131–62. Wiley, Chichester.

Association of Anaesthetists of Great Britain and Ireland (1991). *The high-dependency unit—acute care in the future*. The Association, 9 Bedford Square, London WC1.

Auerbach, S.M. (1973). Trait state anxiety and adjustment to surgery. *Journal of Consulting and Clinical Psychology*, 40(2), 264–71.

Auerbach, S.M. (1979). Preoperative preparation for surgery: a review of recent research and future prospects. In *Research in psychology and medicine*, (ed. D.J. Osborne, M.M. Gruneberg, and J.R. Eiser), Vol. 2: *Social aspects: attitudes, communication, care and training*, pp. 345–9. Academic Press, London.

Auerbach, S.M., Kendall, P.C., Cuttler, H.F., and Leavitt, N.R. (1976). Anxiety, locus of control, type of preparatory information and adjustment to dental surgery. *Journal of Consulting and Clinical Psychology*, 44, 1284–96.

Auerbach, S.M., Martelli, M.F., and Mercuri, I.G. (1983). Anxiety, information, interpersonal impacts, and adjustment to stressful healthcare situation. *Journal of Personality and Social Psychology*, 44, 1284–96.

Austin, K.L., Stapleton, J.V., and Mather, L.E. (1980*a*). Relationship between blood meperidine concentrations and analgesic response. *Anesthesiology*, 53, 460–6.

Austin, K.L., Stapleton, J.V., and Mather, L.E. (1980*b*). Multiple intramuscular injections: a major source of variability in analgesic response to meperidine. *Pain*, 8, 47–62.

Averill, J.R. (1973). Personal control over aversive stimuli and its relationship to stress. *Psychological Bulletin*, 80, 286–303.

Barrier, G. (1985). Requirements for patient controlled analgesia systems. In Patient-controlled analgesia (ed. M. Harmer, M. Rosen, and M.D. Vickers), pp. 81–2. Blackwell Scientific, Oxford.

Beecher, H.K. (1956). Relationship of significance of wound to pain experienced. *Journal of the American Medical Association*, 161, 1609–13.

Belville, J.W., Forrest, W.H., jun., Miller, E., and Brown, B.W. (1971). Influence of age on pain relief from analgesics. *Journal of the American Medical Association*, 217, 1835–41.

Berkowitz, B.A., Ngai, S.H., Yang, J.C., Hampstead, J., and Spector, S. (1975). The disposition of morphine in surgical patients. *Clinical Pharmacology and Therapeutics*, 17, 629–35.

Berlyne, D.E. (1960). *Conflict, arousal and curiosity*. McGraw-Hill, New York.

Bevan, P. (1989). *A study of the management and utilisation of operating departments*. HMSO for the Department of Health, London.

Bond, M.R. (1973). Personality studies in patients with pain secondary to organic disease. *Journal of Psychosomatic Research*, 17, 257.

Bond, M.R. (1978). Psychological and psychiatric aspects of pain. *Anaesthesia*, 33, 355–61.

Bond, M.R. (1981). Personality and pain. In *Persistent pain; Modern methods of treatment*: Vol 2 pp. 1–25 (ed. S. Lipton). Academic Press, London.

Bond, M.R. (1984). *Pain; its nature, analysis, and treatment*. Churchill Livingstone, pp 51–4.

Bone, M.E., Wilkinson, D.J., Young, J.R., McNeil, J., and Charlton, S. (1990). Ginger root—a new antiemetic. The effect of ginger root on postoperative nausea and vomiting after major gynaecological surgery. *Anaesthesia*, 45, 669–71.

Bonilla, K.B., Quigley, W.F., and Bowers, W.F. (1961). Experiences with hypnosis on a surgical service. *Military Medicine*, 126, 364–70.

Boore, J.R.P. (1978). *Information: a prescription for recovery*. Royal College of Nursing, London.

Boyle, P. and Parbrook, G.D. (1977). The interrelation of personality and postoperative factors. *British Journal of Anaesthesia*, 49, 259–63.

Buck, N., Devlin, H.B., and Lunn, J.N. (1989). *Confidential enquiry into perioperative deaths*. Nuffield Provincial Hospitals Trust & King's Fund, London.

Burns, J.W., Hodsman, N.B.A., McLintock, T.T.C., Gillies, G.W.A., Kenny, G.N.C., and McArdle, C.S. (1989). The influence of patient characteristics on the requirements for postoperative analgesia. *Anaesthesia*, 44, 2–6.

Burns, J.W., Aitken, H.A., Bullingham, R.E.S., McArdle, C.S., and Kenny, G.N.C. (1991). Double-blind comparison of the morphine-sparing effect of continuous and intermittent i.m. administration of ketorolac. *British Journal of Anaesthesia*, 67, 235–8.

Byrne, T.J. and Edeani, D. (1983). Knowledge of medical terminology among hospital patients. *Nursing Research*, 33(3), 178–81.

Carnevali, D.L. (1966). Preoperative anxiety. *American Journal of Nursing*, 7, 1536–8.

Cartwright, P.D., Helfinger, R.G., Howell, J.J., and Siepmann, K.K. (1991). Introducing an acute pain service. *Anaesthesia*, 46, 188–91.

Catley, D.M., Thornton, C., Jordan, C., Lehane, J.R., Royston, D., and Jones, J.G. (1985). Pronounced, episodic oxygen desaturation in the postoperative period: its association with ventilatory pattern and analgesic regime. *Anesthesiology*, 63, 20–8.

Catling, J.A., Pinto, D.M., Jordan, C., and Jones, J.G. (1980). Respiratory effects of analgesia after cholecystectomy: comparison of continuous and intermittent papaveretum. *British Medical Journal*, 282, 478–80.

Chapman, C.R. (1984). New directions in the understanding and management of pain. *Journal of Social Science and Medicine*, 19, 1261–77.

Chapman, C.R. and Cox, G.B. (1977). Anxiety, pain and depression surrounding elective surgery: a multivariate comparison of abdominal surgery patients and kidney donors and recipients. *Journal of Psychosomatic Research*, 21, 7–15.

Clark, E., Hodsman, N., and Kenny, G. (1989). Improved postoperative recovery with patient-controlled analgesia. *Nursing Times*, 85, 54–5.

Clum, G.A., Scott, L., and Burnside, J. (1979). Information and locus of control as factors in the outcome of surgery. *Psychological Reports*, 45, 867–73.

Cook, R., Anderson, S., Riseborough, M., and Blogg, C.E. (1990). Intravenous fluid load and recovery. *Anaesthesia*, 45, 826–30.

Cosper, B. (1967). How well do patients understand hospital jargon? *American Journal of Nursing*, 1932–4.

Cromwell, R.L., Butterfield, E.C., Brayfield, F.M., and Curry, J.J. (1977). *Acute myocardial infarction and recovery*. CV Mosby, St Louis.

Cronin, M., Redfern, P.A., and Utting, J.E. (1973). Psychometry and postoperative complaints in surgical patients. *British Journal of Anaesthesia*, 45, 879–86.

Currie, J., Owen, H., Plummer, J.L., and Teitzel, R. (1990). Postoperative PCA with alfentanil. *British Journal of Anaesthesia*, 65, 576P.

Dalrymple, D.G. and Parbrook, G.D. (1976). Personality assessment and postoperative analgesia. *British Journal of Anaesthesia*, 48, 593.

Davies, G.K., Tolhurst-Cleaver, C.L., and James, T.L. (1981). Respiratory depression after intrathecal narcotics. *Anaesthesia*, 36, 268–76.

Davis, B.D. (1984). *Preoperative information-giving and patients' postoperative outcomes*. University of Edinburgh, Department of Nursing Studies.

Davitz, J.R. and Davitz, L.L. (1981). *Inferences of patients' pain and psychological distress: studies of nursing behaviors*. Springer, New York.

Davitz, J.R. and Davitz, L.L. (1985). Culture and nurses' inferences of suffering. In *Perspective on pain* (ed. L. A. Copp), Recent Advances in Nursing Series, 11, pp. 17–28. Churchill Livingstone, Edinburgh.

Dodson, M.E. (1985). *The management of postoperative pain*, Current Topics in Anaesthesia Series, 8. Arnold, London.

Dowie, R. (1991). *Patterns of hospital medical staffing*. Anaesthetics, pp. 46–7. HMSO for the British Postgraduate Medical Federation, London.

Dundee, J.W., Loan, W.B., and Clarke, R.S.J. (1966). Studies of drugs given before anaesthesia. XI diamorphine (heroin) and morphine. *British Journal of Anaesthesia*, 38, 610–19.

Duthie, D., Davies, S.J., and Nimmo, W. (1987). The Travenol infusor. *Care of the critically ill*, 3, no 2.

ECRI (Emergency Care Research Institute) (1988). Evaluation of patient-controlled analgesic infusion pumps. *Health Devices*, 17, 136–67.

Editorial. (1976). Postoperative pain. British Medical Journal 2: 664.

Egbert, L.D., Battitt, G.E., Welch, C.D., and Bartlett, M.K. (1964). Reduction of postoperative pain by encouragement and instructions to patients. *New England Journal of Medicine*, 16, 825–7.

Epstein, S. (1973). Expectancy and magnitude of reaction to noxious UCS. *Psychophysiology* 10, 100–7.

Estok, P.M., Glass, P.S.A., Goldberg, J.S., Freiberger, J.J., and Sladen, R.N. (1987). Use of patient-controlled analgesia to compare intravenous to epidural administration of fentanyl in the postoperative patient. *Anesthesiology*, 67, A230.

Evans, J.M., MacCarthy, J., and Rosen, M. (1976). Apparatus for patient-controlled administration of intravenous narcotics during labour. *Lancet*, 1, 17–18.

Eysenck, H.J. (1967). *The biological basis of personality*. Thomas, Springfield, Illinois.

Farmer, M. and Harper, N.J.N. (1992). Unexpected problems with patient-controlled analgesia. *British Medical Journal*, 304, 574.

Fischberg, B.L., Mead, D.S., and Ritter, H.T.M. (1991). Evaluation and selection of PCA infusion pumps. *Hospital Pharmacy*, 26, 412–23, 451.

Flagherty, G.C. and Fitzpatrick, J.J. (1978). Relaxation technique to increase comfort level of postoperative patients: a preliminary study. *Nursing Research*, 27, 352–5.

Foott, S. (1978). Personal view. *British Medical Journal*, 2, 950.

Fordyce, W.E. (1976). *Behavioural methods for chronic pain and illness*. Mosby, St Louis.

French, K. (1979). Some anxieties of elective surgery patients and the desire for reassurance and information. In *Research in psychological medicine*, Vol.2 (ed. D.J. Osborne, M.M. Gruneberg, and J.R. Eiser, pp. 336–43. Academic Press, New York.

Geer, J.H. and Maisel, E. (1972). Evaluating the effects of prediction control confound. *Journal of Personality and Social Psychology*, 23, 314–19.

Ghaly, R.G., Fitzpatrick, K.T.J., and Dundee, J.W. (1987). Antiemetic studies with traditional Chinese acupuncture. *Anaesthesia*, 42, 1108–10.

Glynn, C.J., Lloyd, J.W., and Folkand, S. (1976). The diurnal variation in the perception of pain. *Proceedings of the Royal Society of Medicine*, 69, 369.

Gould, T.H., Crosby, D.L., Harmer, M. Lloyd, S.M., Lunn, J.N., Rees, G. A.D. *et al.* (1992). Policy for controlling pain after surgery: effect of sequential changes in management. *British Medical Journal*, 305, 1187–93.

Gourlay, G.K., Wilson, P.R., and Glynn, C.J. (1982). Pharmacodynamics and pharmacokinetics of methadone during the perioperative period. *Anesthesiology*, 57, 458.

Graves, D.A., Batenhorst, R.L., Bennett, R.L., Wettstein, J.G., Griffen, W.O., Wright, B.D., *et al.* (1983). Morphine requirements using patient-controlled analgesia: influence of diurnal variation and morbid obesity. *Clinical Pharmacy*, 2, 49–53.

Green, C.P. (1990). The evaluation of pain in man. *Frontiers of pain*, 2, 2.

Grover, E.R. and Heath, M.L. (1992). Patient controlled analgesia: a serious incident. *Anaesthesia*, 47, 402–4.

Hanning, C.D. (1989). Obstructive sleep apnoea. *British Journal of Anaesthesia*, 63, 477–88.

Hanning, C.D. (1992). Prolonged postoperative oxygen therapy. *British Journal of Anaesthesia*, 69, 115–6.

Hartog, J. and Hartog, E.A. (1983). Cultural aspects of health and illness behaviour in hospitals. *Cross cultural medicine. The Western Journal of Medicine*, 139, 910–16.

Haslett, W.H.K. and Dundee, J.W. (1968). Studies of drugs given before anaesthesia. XIV: two benzodiazepine derivatives—chlordiazepoxide and diazepam. *British Journal of Anaesthesia*, 36, 250.

Hayward, J. (1975). *Information: a prescription against pain*, The Study of Nursing Care Reports, Series 2, No. 5. Royal College of Nursing, London.

Heath, M.L. (1992). Learning from someone else's mistakes. *Anaesthesia News*, No. 58 (May 1992).

Henry, J.P. and Stephens, P.M. (1977). *Stress, health and the social environment: a biologic approach*. Springer, New York.

Hester, J.B. and Health, M.L. (1977). Pulmonary acid aspiration syndrome: should prophylaxis be routine? *British Journal of Anaesthesia*, 49, 595–9.

Higgins, M.J., Asbury, A.J., and Brodie, M.J. (1991). Inhaled nebulised fentanyl for postoperative analgesia. *Anaesthesia*, 46, 973–6.

Hill, H.F., Mackie, A.M., Coda, B.A., Iverson, K., and Chapman, C.R. (1991). Patient-controlled analgesic administration. A comparison of steady-state morphine infusions with bolus doses. *Cancer*, 67, 873–82.

Honig, W.J. and Van Ochten, J. (1986). A multiple dose comparison of ketorolac tromethamine with diflunisal and placebo in post-meniscectomy pain. *Journal of Clinical Pharmacology*, 26, 700–5.

Hull, C.J. (1985). The pharmacokinetics of opioid analgesics with special reference to patient-controlled administration. In Patient-controlled analgesia (ed. M. Harmer, M. Rosen, and M.D. Vickers), pp. 7–17. Blackwell Scientific, Oxford.

Hull, C.J. and Sibbald, A. (1981). Control of postoperative pain by interactive demand analgesia. *British Journal of Anaesthesia*, 53, 385–91.

Janis, I.L. (1958). *Psychological stress*. Academic Press, New York.

Johnson, J.E., Leverthal, H, and Dabbs, J.M. (1971). Contribution of emotional and instrumental responses in adaptation to surgery. *Journal of Personality and Social Psychology*, 20, 55–64.

Johnson, J.E. (1973). Effects of accurate expectation about sensations on the sensory and distress components of pain. *Journal of Personality and Social Psychology*, 27, 261–75.

Johnson, J.E. (1983). Preparing patients to cope with stress. In Patient teaching, (ed. J. Wilson-Barnett), Recent Advances in Nursing Series, Vol. 6. Churchill-Livingstone, Edinburgh.

Johnson, T. and Daugherty, M. (1992). Oversedation with patient-controlled analgesia. *Anaesthesia*, 47, 81–2.

Johnson, J.E., Rice, V.H., Fuller, S.S., and Endress, M.P. (1978). Sensory information, instruction in coping strategy and recovery from surgery. *Research in Nursing and Health*, 1, 4–7.

Johnson, L.R., Ferrante, F.M., Magnani, B.J., and Rocco, A.G. (1988). Psychological modifiers of PCA efficacy. *Anaesthesia*, 13, 52S.

Johnston, M. (1980). Anxiety in surgical patients. *Psychological Medicine*, 10, 145–52.

Johnston, M. (1986). Pre-operative emotional states and post-operative recovery. *Advances in psychosomatic medicine*, Vol. 15, 1–22.

Johnston, M. and Carpenter, L. (1980). Relationship between preoperative anxiety and postoperative state. *Psychological Medicine*, 10, 361–7.

Jones, J.A. and Harrop-Griffiths, A.W. (1991). Pain after surgery. *Anaesthesia*, 46, 502–3.

Kaiko, R.F. (1980). Age and morphine analgesia in cancer patients with postoperative pain. *Clinical Pharmacology and Therapeutics*, 28, 823–6.

Kamath, B., Curran, J., Hawkey, C., Beattie, A., Gorbutt, N., Guiblin, H., *et al.* (1990). Anaesthesia, movement and emesis. *British Journal of Anaesthesia*, 64, 728–30.

Kanfer, J.H. and Goldfoot, D.A. (1966). Self-control and the tolerance of noxious stimulation. *Psychological Reports*, 18, 79–85.

Katz, R. and Wykes T., (1985). The psychological difference between temporally predictable and unpredictable stressful events: evidence for informational control theories. *Journal of Personality and Social Psychology*, 48, 781–90.

Kay, N.H., Allen, M.C., Bullingham, R.E.S., Baldwin, D., McQuay, R.J., Moore, H.A., *et al.* (1985). Influence of meptazinol on metabolic and hormonal responses following major surgery. A comparison with morphine. *Anaesthesia*, 40, 223–8.

Kendall, P.C., Williams, L., Perchacek, T.F., Graham, L.E. Shisslak, C., and Herzoff, N. (1979). Cognitive-behavioural and patient-education interventions in cardiac catheterization procedures. *Journal of Consulting and Clinical Psychology*, 47, 49–58.

Khun, S., Cooke, K., Collins, M., Jones, J.M., and Mucklow, J.C. (1990). Perceptions of pain relief after surgery. *British Medical Journal*, 300, 1687–90.

Klos, D., Cummings, M., Joyce, J., *et al.* (1980). A comparison of two methods of delivering presurgical information. *Patient Counselling and Health*, Education, 1, 6–13.

Kluger, M.T. and Owen, H. (1990). Patients' expectations of patient-controlled analgesia. *Anaesthesia*, 45, 1072–4.

Kluger, M.T. and Owen, H. (1991). On-demand epidural fentanyl. *Anaesthesia*, 46, 983–4.

Kolouch, F.T. (1964). Hypnosis and surgical convalescence. *American Journal of Clinical Hypnotherapy*, 7, 120–9.

Kornfield, D.S., Heller, S.S., Frank, K.A., and Moskowitz, R. (1974). Personality and psychological factors in post-cardiotomy delirium. *Archives of General Psychiatry*, 31, 249–53.

Langer, E.J., Janis, I., and Wolfer, J. (1975). Reduction of psychological stress in surgical patients. *Journal of Experimental and Social Psychology*, 11, 155–65.

Lazarus, R.S. (1966). *Psychological stress and the coping process.* McGraw Hill, New York.

Lim, A.T., Edis, G., Kranz, H., Mendleson, G., Selwood, T., and Scott, D.F. (1983). Postoperative pain control: contribution of psychological factors and transcutaneous electrical stimulation. *Pain*, 17, 179–88.

Lindeman, C.A. and Van Aernam, B. (1971). Nursing intervention with presurgical patients; the effects of structures and unstructured preoperative teaching. *Nursing Research*, 20, 319–32.

Lipton, J. and Marbach, J. (1984). Ethnicity in pain experience. *Social Science and Medicine*, 19, 1279–98.

Lloyd-Thomas, A.R. (1990). Pain management in paediatric patients. *British Journal of Anaesthesia*, 64, 85–103.

Loo, R. (1979). Note on the relationship between trait anxiety and Eysenck personality questionnaire. *Journal of Clinical Psychology*, 35, 110.

Lunn, J.N. and Mushin, W.W. (1982). *Mortality associated with anaesthesia.* Nuffield Provincial Hospitals Trust, London.

McQuay, H. (1988). Potential problems of using both opioids and local anaesthetic. *British Journal of Anaesthesia*, 61, 121.

McQuay, H. (1992). Pre-emptive analgesia. *British Journal of Anaesthesia*, 69, 1–3.

McQuay, H.J., Poppleton, P., Carroll, D., Summerfield, R.J., Bullingham, R.E.S., and Moore, R.E. (1986). Ketorolac and acetaminophen for orthopaedic postoperative pain. *Clinical Pharmacology and Therapeutics*, 39, 89–93.

Madej, T.H., Wheatley, R.G., Jackson, I.J.B., Hunter, D. (1992). Hypoxaemia and pain relief after lower abdominal surgery: comparison of extradural and patient-controlled analgesia. *British Journal of Anaesthesia*, 69, 554–7.

Maltby, J.R., Ewen, A., Koehli, N., and Strunin, L. (1988). Preoperative fluids, ranitidine and opiate-atropine premedication. *British Journal of Anaesthesia*, 61, 113–114P.

Mandler, G. (1972). Helplessness: theory and research in anxiety. In Anxiety, current trends in theory and research (ed. C. D. Spielberger), pp. Academic Press, New York.

Mandler, G. and Watson, D.L. (1966). Anxiety and the interruption of behaviour. In Anxiety and behaviour (ed. C. D. Spielberger), pp. 263–90. Academic Press, New York.

Marshall, B.E. and Wyche, M. (1972). Hypoxemia during and after anesthesia. *Anesthesiology* 37, 178–209.

Martinez-Urrutia, A. (1975). Anxiety and pain in surgical patients. *Journal of Consulting and Clinical Psychology*, 43, 437–42.

Mather, L.E. (1983). Pharmacokinetic and pharmacodynamic factors influencing the choice, dose and route of administration of opiates for acute pain. *Clinics in Anaesthesiology*, Vol. 1 no. 1, 17–41.

Mather, L.E. and Mackie, J. (1983). The incidence of postoperative pain in children. *Pain*, 15, 271–82.

Mathews, A. and Ridgeway, V. (1981). Personality and surgical recovery. *British Journal of Clinical Psychology*, 20, 243–60.

Maynard, A. (1987). Logic in medicine: an economic perspective. *British Medical Journal*, 295, 1537–41.

Melzack, R. (1975). The McGill Pain Questionnaire: major properties and scoring methods. *Pain*, 1, 275–99.

Melzack, R. (1987). The short form McGill Pain Questionnaire. *Pain*, 30, 191–7.

Melzack, R. and Wall, P.D. (1965). Pain mechanisms: a new theory. *Science*, 150, 971–9.

Melzack, R. and Wall, P.D. (1988). *The challenge of pain.* Penguin Books, London.

Migliore, S. (1989). Punctuality, pain and time-orientation amongst Sicilian-Canadians. *Social Science and Medicine,* 28, 851–9.

Miller, S.M. (1979). Controllability and human stress: method, evidence and theory. *Behaviour Research and Theory,* 17, 287–304.

Miller, S.M. (1980). When is a little information a dangerous thing? Coping with stressful life events by monitoring vs blunting. In *Coping and Health,* (ed. S. Levine and H. Ursin), pp. 145–69. Plenum Press, New York.

Miller, S.M. (1981). Predictability and human stress: towards a clarification of evidence and theory. In Advances in experimental social psychology, Vol. 14 (ed. L. Berkowitz), pp. Academic Press, New York.

Miller, S.M. (1987). Monitoring and blunting: validation of a questionnaire to assess different styles for coping with stress. *Journal of Personality and Social Psychology,* 52, 345–53.

Miller, S.M. and Mangan, C.E. (1983). The interacting effects of information and coping style in adapting to gynaecologic stress. *Journal of Personality and Social Psychology,* 45, 223–36.

Miller, J.F. and Shuter, R. (1984). Age, sex and race affect pain expression. *American Journal of Nursing,* Aug. 1984, 981.

Miller, M., Wishart, H.Y., and Nimmo, W.S. (1983). Gastric contents at induction of anaesthesia; is a four hour fast necessary? *British Journal of Anaesthesia,* 55, 1185–8.

Mills, G.H. and Goddard, J.M. (1991). A case of patient-controlled analgesia exacerbating postoperative pain. *Anaesthesia,* 46, 893.

Mitchell, A., Brunner, M., Fisher, A.P., Ware, R.G., and Hanna, M. (1991). Pethidine for painful crises in sickle cell disease. *British Medical Journal,* 303, 249.

Monat, A., Averill, J.R., and Lazarus, R.G. (1972). Anticipator, stress and coping reactions under various conditions of uncertainty. *Journal of Personality and Social Psychology,* 24, 237–53.

Morrison, L.M., Payne, M., and Drummond, G.P. (1991). Comparison of speed of onset of analgesic effect of diamorphine and morphine. *British Journal of Anaesthesia,* 66, 656–9.

Mowbray, M.J. and Gaukroger, P.B. (1990). Long-term patient-controlled analgesia in children. *Anaesthesia,* 45, 941–3.

Nayman, J. (1979). Measurement and control of postoperative pain. *Annals of the Royal College of Surgeons,* 61, 419.

Nolan, K.M., Baxter, M.K., Winyard, J.A., Roulson, C.J., and Goldhill, D.R. (1992). Video surveillance of oxygen administration by mask in postoperative patients. *British Journal of Anaesthesia,* 69, 194–6.

Notcutt, W.G. and Morgan, R.J.M. (1990). Introducing PCA for postoperative pain control into a DGH. *Anaesthesia,* 45, 401–6.

Notcutt, W.G., Knowles, P., and Kaldas, R. (1992). Overdose of opioid from patient-controlled analgesia pumps. *British Journal of Anaesthesia*, 69, 95–7.

Nunn, J.F. and Payne, J.P. (1962). Hypoxaemia after general anaesthesia, *Lancet* ii 631–4.

Owen, H., Glavin, R.J., Reekie, R.M., and Trew, A.S. (1986). Patient-controlled analgesia. Experience of two new machines. *Anaesthesia*, 41, 1230–5.

Owen, H., Szerkely, S.M., Plummer, J.L., Cushnie, J.M., and Mather, L.E. (1989). Variables of patient-controlled analgesia: 2. Concurrent infusion. *Anaesthesia*, 44, 11–13.

Owens, J.F. and Hutlemeyer, C.M. (1982). The effect of pre-operative intervention on delirium in cardiac surgical patients. Nursing Research, 31, 60–2.

Palazzo, M.G.A. and Strunin, L. (1984). Anaesthesia and emesis 1: etiology. *Canadian Anaesthetists' Society Journal*, 31, 178–87.

Parker, R.K., Holmann, B., Woodring-Brown, P., and White, P.F. (1989). Effects of a basal opioid infusion on the postoperative analgesic requirement. *Anesthesiology*, 71, A763.

Peck, C.L. (1986). Psychological factors in acute pain management. In Acute pain management (ed. M.J. Cousins and G.D. Phillips), pp. 251–74. Churchill Livingstone, Edinburgh.

Pendleton, D. and Bochner, S. (1980). The communication of medical information in general practice consultations as a function of patients' social class. *Social Science and Medicine*, 14A, 669–73.

Pickett, C. and Clum, G.A. (1982). Comparative treatment strategies and their interaction with locus of control in the reduction of postsurgical pain and anxiety. *Journal of Consulting and Clinical Psychology*, 50, 439–41.

Pleuvry, B.J. (1991). Opioid receptors and their ligands: natural and unnatural. *British Journal of Anaesthesia*, 66, 370–80.

Popat, M.T., Dyar, O.J., and Blogg, C.E. (1991). Comparison of the effects of oral nizatidine and ranitidine on gastric volume in patients undergoing gynaecological laparoscopy. *Anaesthesia*, 46, 816–19.

Porter, J. and Jick, H. (1979). Addiction rare in patients treated with narcotics. *New England Journal of Medicine*, 302, 123.

Pryle, B.J., Grech, H., Stoddart, P.A., Carson, R., O'Mahoney, T., and Reynolds, F. (1992). Toxicity of norpethidine in sickle cell crisis. *British Medical Journal*, 304, 1478–9.

Reading, A.E. (1984). Testing pain mechanisms in persons in pain. In Textbook of pain (ed. P.D. Wall and R. Melzack), pp. 195–206. Churchill Livingstone, Edinburgh.

Reeder, M.K., Goldman, M.D., Loh, L., Muir, A.D., Casey, K.R., and Gitlin, D.A. (1991a). Postoperative obstructive sleep apnoea, haemodynamic effects of treatment with nasal CPAP. *Anaesthesia*, 46, 849–53.

Reeder, M.K., Muir, A.D., Foex, P., Goldman, M.D., Loh, L., and Smart,

D. (1991*b*). Postoperative myocardial ischaemia: temporal association with nocturnal hypoxaemia. *British Journal of Anaesthesia*, 67, 626–31.

Ridgeway, V. and Mathews, A. (1982). Psychological preparation for surgery: a comparison of methods. *British Journal of Clinical Psychology*, 21, 271–80.

Robinson, S.L., Rowbotham, D.J., and Smith, G. (1991). Morphine compared with diamorphine. A comparison of dose requirements and side effects after hip surgery. *Anaesthesia*, 46, 538–40.

Rogers, M. and Reich, P. (1986). Psychological intervention with surgical patients: outcome evaluation. *Advances in Psychosomatic Medicine*, 15, 23–50.

Rosenberg, J., Dirkes, W.E., and Kehlet, H. (1989). Episodic arterial oxygen desaturation and heart rate variations following major abdominal surgery. *British Journal of Anaesthesia*, 63, 651–4.

Rowbotham, D.J., Wyld, R., and Nimmo, W.S. (1989*a*) A disposable device for PCA with fentanyl. *Anaesthesia*, 44, 922–4.

Rowbotham, D.J., Wyld, R., Peacock, J.E., Duthie, D.J.R., and Nimmo, W.S. (1989*b*) Transdermal fentanyl for the relief of pain after upper abdominal surgery. *British Journal of Anaesthesia*, 63, 56–9.

Royal College of Surgeons and College of Anaesthetists. Joint Working Party (1990). *Pain after surgery*. Report of a working party of the Commission on the Provision of Services. The Colleges, London.

Schorr, D. and Rodin, J. (1984). Motivation to control one's environment in individuals with obsessive compulsive, depressive, and normal personality traits. *Journal of Personality and Social Psychology*, 46, 1148–61.

Scott, J. and Huskisson, E.C. (1976). Graphic representation of pain. *Pain*, 2, 175–84.

Scott, L.E., Clum, G.A., and Peoples, J.B. (1983). Preoperative predictors of postoperative pain. *Pain*, 15, 283–93.

Sechzer, P.H. (1968). Objective measurement of pain. *Anesthesiology*, 29, 209–10.

Seers, C.J. (1987). Pain anxiety and recovery in patients undergoing surgery. Ph. D. thesis, University of London.

Seligman, M.E.P. (1975). *Helplessness*. Freeman Press, San Francisco.

Seligman, M., Maier, S., and Soloman, R. (1971). Unpredictable and uncontrollable aversive events. In: *Aversive conditioning and learning* (ed. F. R. Brush). Academic Press, New York.

Seymour, R.A. (1982). The use of pain scales in assessing the efficacy of analgesics in postoperative dental pain. *European Journal of Clinical Pharmacology*, 23, 441–4.

Smith, L.S. (1974). An investigation of pre- and postsurgical anxiety as a function of relaxation training. Doctoral dissertation, University of South Missisippi, Hattiesburg.

Smith, M.B. and Elwood, R.J. (1988). Patient-controlled analgesia. *Anaesthesia*, 43, 802–3.

Spielberger, C.D., Auerbach, S.M., Wadsworth, A., Dumm, T.M., and Taulbee, S.M. (1973). Emotional reactions to surgery. *Journal of Consulting and Clinical Psychology*, 40, 33–8.

Stack, C.G. and Massey, N.J. (1990). Bradypnoea during patient-controlled analgesia. *Anaesthesia*, 45, 683–4.

Sternbach, R.A. (1968). Pain: a psychological analysis. Academic Press, New York.

Sternbach, R.A. (1978). The psychology of pain. Raven Press, New York.

Streltzer, J. and Wade, T.C. (1981). The influence of cultural group on the undertreatment of postoperative pain. *Psychosomatic Medicine*, 43, 397.

Surnam, O.S., Hacket, T.P., Silverberg, E.L., et al. (1974). Usefulness of psychiatric intervention in patients undergoing cardiac surgery. *Archives of General Psychiatry*, 30, 830–5.

Taenzer, P.A., Melzack, R., and Jeans, M.E. (1986). Influence of psychological factors on postoperative pain, mood and analgesic requirements. *Pain*, 24, 331–42.

Taylor, J.A. (1953). A personality scale of manifest anxiety. *Journal of Abnormal and Social Psychology*, 48, 285–90.

Taylor, D.M. and Heath, M.L. (1992). A disposable device for patient-controlled analgesia compared to intramuscular papaveretum. *Hospital Pharmacy Practice*, 2, 623–8.

Taylor, T.H., Jennings, A.M.C., Nightingale, D.A., Barker, B., Leivers, D., Styles, M., et al. (1969). A study of anaesthetic emergency work. Paper I: The method of study and introduction to queuing theory. *British Journal of Anaesthesia*, 41, 70–5.

Teillol-Foo, W.L.M. (1991). Indwelling intramuscular cannula for postoperative analgesia. *Anaesthesia*, 46, 897.

Thomas, V.J. (1991). Personality characteristics of patients and the effectiveness of P.C.A. Unpublished Ph.D. thesis. Goldsmith's College, University of London.

Thomas, V.J. and Rose, D. (1991). Ethnic differences in the experience of pain. *Social Science and Medicine*, 32, 1063–6.

Thomas, V.J., Heath, M.L., and Rose, F.D. (1990). Effect of psychological variables and pain relief system on postoperative pain experience. *British Journal of Anaesthesia*, 64, 388P–389P.

Thompson, S.C. (1981). Will it hurt less if I can control it? A complex answer to a simple question. *Psychological Bulletin*, 90, 89–101.

Thomsen, K.A., Terkildsen, K., and Arnfred, I. (1965). Middle ear pressure variations during nitrous oxide and oxygen anaesthesia. *Archives of Otolaryngology*, 82, 609–11.

Tverskoy, M., Cozacov, C., Ayache, M., Bradley, E.L., and Kissin, I. (1990). Postoperative pain after inguinal herniorraphy with different types of anesthesia. *Anesthesia and Analgesia*, 70, 29–35.

References 211

Vernon, D.T.A. and Bigelow, D.A. (1974). Effect of information about a potentially stressful situation on response to impact. *Journal of Personality and Social Psychology*, 29, 50–9.

Welchew, E.A. (1983). On-demand analgesia. A double blind comparison of on-demand intravenous fentanyl with regular intramuscular morphine. *Anaesthesia*, 38, 19–25.

Welchew, E.A. (1991a). On demand epidural fentanyl: a reply (a). *Anaesthesia*, 46, 984.

Welchew, E.A. (1991b). On demand epidural fentanyl: a reply (b). *Anaesthesia*, 46, 985.

Welchew, E.A. and Breen, D.P. (1991). Patient-controlled on-demand epidural fentanyl. A comparison of patient-controlled on-demand fentanyl delivered epidurally or intravenously. *Anaesthesia*, 46, 438–41.

Wells, J.K., Howard, G.S., Nowlin, W.F., and Vargas, M.J. (1986). Presurgical anxiety and postsurgical pain and adjustment. *Journal of Consulting and Clinical Psychology*, 54, 831–5.

Wheatley, R.G., Madej, T.H., Jackson, I.J.B., and Hunter, D. (1991). The first year's experience of an acute pain service. *British Journal of Anaesthesia*, 67, 353–9.

Wheatley, R.G., Somerville, I.D., Sapsford, D.J., and Jones, J.G. (1990). Postoperative hypoxaemia: comparison of extradural, IM and patient-controlled opioid analgesia. *British Journal of Anaesthesia*, 64, 267–75.

Wheatley, R.G., Shepherd, D., Jackson, I.J.B., Madej, T.H., Hunter, D. (1992). Hypoxaemia and pain relief after upper abdominal surgery: comparison of i.m. and patient-controlled analgesia. *British Journal of Anaesthesia*, 69, 558–61.

Williams, O.A., Clarke, F.L., Harris, R.W., Smith, P., and Peacock, J.E. (1993). Addition of droperidol to patient controlled analgesia: effect on nausea and vomiting. British Journal of Anaesthesia, 70, 479P.

Wilson, J.F. (1981). Behavioural preparation for surgery: benefit or harm? *Journal of Behavioural Medicine*, Vol. 4, 79–102.

Wilson, J.F. and Bennett, R.L. (1984). Coping styles, medication use and pain scores in patients using PCA for postoperative pain. *Anesthesiology*, 61, A193.

Wilson-Barnett, J. (1979). Stress in hospital: patients' psychological reactions to hospitalization. Churchill Livingstone, Edinburgh.

Wilson-Barnett, J. (1988). Anxiety. In *Patients' problems: a research base for nursing care* (ed. J. Wilson-Barnett and Batehup), pp. 31–57; Scutari Press.

Wolfer, J.A. and Davis, C.E. (1970). Assessment of patients' preoperative emotional condition and postoperative welfare. *Nursing Research*, 19, 402–14.

Woodrow, K.M., Friedman, G.D., Siegelbaub, A.B., and Collen, M.F. (1972). Pain tolerance: differences according to age, sex and race. *Psychosomatic Medicine*, 34, 548.

Yaksh, T.L., Al-Rodhan, N.R.F., and Mjanger, E. (1988). Sites of action of opiates in production of analgesia. In Anaesthesia Review 5 (ed. L. Kaufman), pp. 254–68. Churchill Livingstone, Edinburgh.

Zborowski, M. (1952). Cultural components in responses to pain. *Journal of Social Issues*, **8**, 16–30.

Zeimer, M.M. (1983). Effects of information on postsurgical coping. *Nursing Research*, **32**, 282–7.

Index